Teenagers with Obesity: How Overweight Kids and Teenagers Can Develop Healthy Habits to Thrive and Live Their Life in Full

By

Karen F. Villa

Copyright and Disclaimer for "Teenagers with Obesity: How Overweight Kids and Teenagers Can Develop Healthy Habits to Thrive and Live Their Life in Full."

This book is intended for general informational purposes only and does not constitute professional advice. The author and publisher assume no responsibility for errors or omissions and disclaim any liability, loss, or risk incurred as a consequence of the use and application, directly or indirectly, of any information presented in this book.

The author is not a licensed healthcare provider, and the content of this book should not be considered a substitute for professional medical, psychological, or nutritional advice, diagnosis, or treatment. Readers are advised to consult with appropriate professionals for specific advice tailored to their individual situations.

Any resemblance to actual persons, living or dead, events, or locales is entirely coincidental.

While every effort has been made to ensure the accuracy and completeness of the information presented, the author and publisher do not warrant or represent that the contents are accurate, reliable, or current. The inclusion of any links does not necessarily imply a recommendation or endorsement of the views expressed within them.

By reading this book, the reader acknowledges and agrees to the terms of this copyright and disclaimer.

About the Author: Karen F. Villa

Mother and Proponent of Positive Living.

Karen F. Villa is a devoted mother whose work skillfully combines advocacy for positive, healthy living with her own experience. Her broadly based articles inspire families to prioritize well-being and adopt healthy lifestyle modifications. Beyond books, Karen actively engages communities to create a supportive atmosphere that helps people and families on their path to a happy and full existence.

Table of Content

Introduction

The problem of obesity can be a distraction from the colourful experiences that should characterise this life-changing stage of adolescence, a time when bodies are changing and hormones are soaring. Adolescent obesity is a rising global health concern that involves more than just physical obesity. It is a multifaceted condition affecting a teen's emotional, social, and physical health.

Teens wrestle with their identities, try to fit in, and long for acceptance throughout the self-discovery phase of adolescence. Due to the stigma and negative connotations attached to obesity, it can undermine one's self-worth and cause feelings of loneliness, anxiety, and sadness. A vicious loop that undermines their general wellbeing can be initiated by the weight of these emotional loads, which can worsen poor eating habits.

Beyond the psychological costs, obesity puts teenagers' health at serious risk. Their developing bodies are strained by the extra weight, which raises their chance of chronic illnesses including diabetes, heart disease, and some types of cancer. Far from being remote threats, these health issues might show up as weariness, decreased mobility, and a general decline in quality of life.

Teenage obesity has become an urgent worry at a time of changing social standards and a broad range of lifestyles.

This book's title, "Teenagers with Obesity: How Overweight Kids and Teenagers Can Develop Healthy Habits to Thrive and Live Their Life in Full," sums up its goal beyond just identifying obesity as a health problem. It represents a call to action for a comprehensive change that prioritises the emotional and psychological fulfilment of teenagers dealing with the difficulties of obesity in addition to their physical well-being.

Teenage obesity is a complex problem that is impacted by lifestyle, environmental, and hereditary factors. The effects include mental health, self-worth, and general quality of life in addition to physical health. Understanding how difficult this task is, the book aims to provide more than just standard weight-loss guidance. This manual was created with the goal of fostering enduring

Understanding how difficult this task is, the book aims to provide more than just standard weight-loss guidance. It's a manual designed to help overweight teenagers create healthy habits, accept who they are, and set out on a path to success in all facets of their lives. The goal is to inspire long-lasting change in these youngsters.

This project is urgent because of the widespread emphasis on appearance in society and the possible long-term effects of obesity. In contrast to maintaining impractical benchmarks, the book proposes a paradigm change. It challenges readers to change their attention from the limited objective of losing weight to the more general one of achieving total well-being. The book seeks to address emotional eating patterns, promote healthy lifestyle choices, and comprehend the underlying reasons of obesity. The book aims to empower teenagers to live their lives to the fullest.

"Live Their Life in Full" perfectly captures the spirit of the book. Beyond just a physical change, it represents the idea of accepting one's actual self free from social pressures. In order to inspire youth to adopt healthy behaviours, the book offers a thorough approach that emphasises sustainable practices, gradual adjustments, and an emphasis on overall well-being rather than weight loss alone. It emphasises the importance of getting professional help when necessary and highlights the role that dietitians, therapists, and paediatricians play in offering individualised care.

The goal of this book is to encourage teens, their families, and communities to overcome the obstacles of obesity and adopt a better lifestyle through anthologies, professional insights, and helpful advice. It imagines a world in which strong and self-assured youth can live life to the fullest, unburdened by the stigma of obesity and open to the countless opportunities that lie ahead.

The Purpose of this Book

"Teenagers with Obesity: How Overweight Kids and Teenagers Can Develop Healthy Habits to Thrive and Live Their Life in Full," is an extensive book that offers teens dealing with obesity difficulties a route towards wellbeing.

This book's goal goes well beyond helping readers lose weight; it's a comprehensive guide that encourages teens to adopt a healthy lifestyle, improving their social, mental, and physical health. It acknowledges that obesity is a complicated web of interrelated elements that can have a substantial impact on a person's general health and happiness rather than just being a medical problem.

This book is based on a profound awareness of the social and emotional toll that teenage obesity takes. Teenagers struggle with emotions of loneliness, anxiety, and despair in a world that stigmatizes obesity, which encourages them to continue bad eating habits. In order to foster a supportive and empowering environment where teenagers feel empowered to make wise decisions, this book promotes empathy, compassion, and a nonjudgmental attitude.

The complex interactions between heredity, environment, and lifestyle choices are examined as the book dives into the fundamental causes of obesity. It busts popular fallacies and misunderstandings, highlighting the significance of tailored approaches that take into account each teen's particular situation.

The idea that adopting a healthier lifestyle is about more than just losing weight is a major component of this book. It includes forming enduring routines, fostering self-acceptance, and placing an emphasis on one's general wellbeing. The book offers helpful advice on how to deal with emotional eating behaviors, incorporate fun physical activities, and encourage gradual adjustments.

It is stressed throughout the book how important it is to get competent advice. In order to provide each adolescent with individualised support that meets their unique needs and makes sure that their emotional and social wellbeing is not disregarded, paediatricians, nutritionists, and therapists are essential.

Beyond just inspiring kids, the book is also a great resource for their families and communities. It offers advice on how to build an encouraging atmosphere at home, encourage candid communication, and recognize small accomplishments. It inspires societies to adopt inclusive behaviours and combat the stigmas attached to obesity.

One of the main goals of the book is to demolish the stigma attached to obesity in teenagers. Teens who are obese are marginalised as a result of society's frequent upholding of unattainable beauty standards. The book aims to promote resilience and self-acceptance by highlighting the intrinsic value of every person, regardless of weight. This goal goes beyond what is written in the book; it is to start a positive chain reaction that affects communities, families, and the larger public conversation around adolescent health. It imagines a day where all teenagers, no matter how big or small, are able to experience life to the fullest and prosper.

In the end, this book offers teens struggling with obesity a ray of hope by showing them the way to happier and healthier lives. It is evidence of the resiliency and potential of teenagers, showing that they can flourish and seize all of life's opportunities with the right help, guidance, and decisions.

Chapter One: Understanding Teen Obesity

A complete approach that takes into account not just physical health but also emotional, social, and psychological well-being is necessary to comprehend teen obesity, an increasing global epidemic. Obesity can be a major concern during adolescence, a time of self-discovery when teens strive to accept their new identities and deal with their changing bodies.

Because obesity is frequently stigmatised and linked to unfavourable opinions, it can lower self-esteem and cause feelings of loneliness, anxiety, and despair. Their overall wellbeing may be hampered by a vicious cycle of bad eating habits made worse by the weight of these emotional problems.

A comprehensive strategy is needed to combat teen obesity, one that abandons the deficit-based model of restriction and shame in favor of a caring and encouraging environment that gives adolescents the freedom to choose wisely and adopt a wholesome lifestyle. In light of the interaction of genetics, environment, and lifestyle variables, this change necessitates a greater comprehension of the underlying causes of obesity.

Metabolism and appetite control are two aspects of obesity that are influenced by genetic predisposition. On the other hand, these genetic predispositions are highly influenced by lifestyle and environmental circumstances. Teenage obesity is becoming more common, and the causes include an excess of processed foods, a decline in physical exercise, and an increase in screen time.

A comprehensive strategy addressing these environmental and behavioral factors is necessary to combat teen obesity. This entails fostering a healthy diet, motivating consistent exercise, and forming sound sleeping practices. It is imperative to acknowledge that these modifications have to be gradual and enduring, conforming to the adolescent's inclinations and way of living.

1. Causes of Obesity and Contributing Factors

1. Genetic Proneness

Obesity in children and adolescents is largely influenced by genetic predispositions. Dispelling falsehoods, lowering stigma, and guiding successful therapies all depend on an understanding of the complex genetic shade that underlies vulnerability to obesity.

Genetic predispositions do not dictate a person's destiny, even though they do pave the way for obesity. The manifestation of these inherited traits can be strongly Influenced by lifestyle choices, particularly those related to nutrition and physical activity. Genetic predispositions can be lessened by leading a healthy lifestyle, but their effects can be increased by making poor decisions.

Understanding how genes and environment interact opens the door to a more individualized and caring approach to treating childhood and adolescent obesity, resulting in a healthier future for future generations. The tendency for obesity in an individual is mostly shaped by genetics. The higher incidence of obesity in family members, which suggests a weight growth pattern passed down through the generations, is indicative of this genetic tendency. Almost 800 genes have been linked to obesity in studies, and these genes affect things like energy metabolism, distribution of fat, and appetite control.

A prominent illustration is the FTO gene, which seems to affect a person's sensitivity to hormones that control hunger and energy expenditure. Differences in this gene have been associated with a higher risk of obesity, especially when paired with bad lifestyle choices. Likewise, the regulation of appetite and food intake is significantly influenced by the MC4R gene. This gene can get mutated to cause monogenic obesity, a disorder marked by significant obesity that develops early in life.

Genetic changes that are inherited can affect the body's ability to store and use energy, as well as how it regulates hunger and metabolism. Even though genes don't work in a vacuum, they do influence how a person reacts to external cues, which makes some people more susceptible to problems related to weight than others.

Several investigations have pinpointed particular genetic markers linked to obesity. Genes involved in energy expenditure, fat metabolism, and appetite regulation have polymorphisms that affect an individual's risk of obesity. Knowing these genetic foundations helps explain why some kids and teens could have a harder time keeping up a healthy weight even with comparable environmental exposures.

One gene or one genetic mutation is not the only factor that affects how obesity risk is inherited. Instead, it is the result of a complicated interaction between several genes, each of which has a subtle effect on different facets of energy balance and metabolism. This polygenic character emphasizes the need for a more complex understanding than the oversimplified concepts of "obesity genes." It entails understanding the complex network of genetic interactions that, when combined, they can collectively shape an individual's propensity for obesity.

It is essential to comprehend genetic predispositions as contributors to obesity and as its causes for two main reasons.

Primarily, it encourages a departure from stigmatizing viewpoints that ascribe obesity only to lifestyle decisions. Acknowledging the hereditary component highlights the fact that people's weight destiny is shaped by natural forces outside their control, rather than just them. In order to combat childhood and teenage obesity, this change in perspective is essential for developing empathy and compassion.

Secondly, customized treatments are informed by the recognition of genetic predispositions. More focused and efficient methods of managing weight are possible when strategies are customized according to a person's genetic profile. The creation of individualized diet plans, fitness schedules, and behavioral interventions can be guided by genetic information, increasing the likelihood of success in the fight against obesity.

2. Environmental Factors

Although genetic predispositions unquestionably contribute to weight control, an individual's propensity to obesity is greatly influenced by environmental variables. Gaining a thorough understanding of these environmental elements and how they affect weight control is necessary to effectively address this issue.

The contemporary food scene is dominated by processed meals, which are frequently loaded with added sugar, bad fats, and excessive calories. Due to their widespread marketing and ease of access, these foods have normalized themselves into everyday diets, which has led to overindulgence and weight gain. Consumption of complete, unprocessed meals including fruits, vegetables, and whole grains declines as a result of the price and convenience of processed foods, which frequently outweighs their nutritious benefit. This change in eating habits upsets the body's normal nutrient balance, which causes an energy imbalance that encourages weight growth.

One of the main environmental factors contributing to obesity in children and teenagers is a marked decrease in physical activity. There are several reasons for this pattern, including:

Increased Screen Time: Sedentary behaviors have increased as a result of the ubiquitous presence of technology, especially screen time spent on computers, smartphones, and televisions. These pursuits lower levels of physical activity and exacerbate energy imbalances.

Sedentary Lifestyles: Modern lives frequently prioritize tasks requiring little physical effort, such driving, taking public transportation, and studying. This inactivity raises the risk of obesity and decreases energy expenditure.

Limited Opportunities for Safe Outdoor Play: Children's and teenagers' access to safe outdoor play areas has been reduced due to urbanization and the loss of open spaces. A further factor in the decline in physical activity is the absence of access to secure recreational areas.

Particularly for kids and teenagers, societal standards and marketing strategies have a big impact on what they eat and how active they are. Unhealthy eating habits are encouraged by the abundance of fast food, sugary drinks, and unhealthy snacks that are readily available in convenience stores, schools, and vending machines.

Additionally, deceptive advertising campaigns aimed at kids and teenagers frequently glorify processed foods and inactive lifestyles while promoting unrealistic body standards that can worsen body image issues and discourage exercise.

Teenagers' and children's vulnerability to obesity is influenced by socioeconomic and family aspects as well. Secure leisure areas and fresh, healthful foods may be more difficult for families with low incomes to access. Moreover, children's choices and behaviors might be influenced by the food and exercise habits of their parents.

Children's and teenagers' predisposition to obesity is greatly influenced by their environment. Effective obesity prevention and lifetime health promotion can be achieved by targeting these factors with comprehensive interventions that support physical activity, good eating, and oppose detrimental influences.

3. Way of Life Decisions

Being overweight affects both adults and children worldwide and is a complicated, multifaceted problem. Genes certainly have an impact, but lifestyle decisions—especially those related to nutrition and exercise—have a significant impact on a person's risk of obesity. It takes a thorough grasp of these lifestyle factors and how they affect weight management to properly address this issue.

1. Nutritional Practices: The Cornerstone of Well-Being Weight Management

A person's weight status is mostly determined by their dietary choices. Eating a diet high in fruits, vegetables, and whole grains and low in processed foods and sugar-filled beverages will help you maintain a healthy weight and control your calorie intake.

But contemporary lifestyles frequently encourage a diet that is typified by:

Overdosing on Calories: Processed foods are widely available and are high in calories, bad fats, and sugar. This leads to overindulgence and weight gain. These meals, which are widely accessible and frequently promoted, give off rapid energy but are deficient in important nutrients, which might cause an imbalance in energy levels.

Poor Nutritional Decisions: When the body doesn't get enough whole, unprocessed meals like fruits, vegetables, and whole grains, it loses out on vital elements like fiber, vitamins, and minerals. These nutrients are essential for maintaining general health, controlling metabolism, and encouraging fullness.

Sugary Drink Consumption: Sugary drinks, such as juices, sodas, and coffee beverages with added sugar, greatly increase the amount of calories consumed in excess, especially for kids and teenagers. These beverages increase the risk of developing chronic illnesses and deliver empty calories devoid of vital nutrients, which can cause weight gain.

2. Engaging in Physical Activity: Improving Energy Use and General Health

Keeping a healthy weight and enhancing general wellbeing require regular physical activity. Consistent physical activity can be promoted by taking part in pleasurable and sustainable activities, which can improve general health and lower the risk of obesity.

But adults' and children's levels of physical activity have drastically decreased, which has contributed to the obesity pandemic. There are several reasons for this pattern, including:

Sedentary Ways of Living: Activities that need little physical effort, like studying, working at a desk, and using technology, are frequently preferred in modern lifestyles.

This inactivity raises the risk of obesity and decreases energy expenditure.

Decreased Emphasis on Physical Education: As physical education has received less attention in schools, there are fewer opportunities for kids to participate in regular physical activity and form good habits that will last a lifetime.

Restricted Access to Recreational Spaces: As a result of societal urbanization and the loss of open spaces, there is a reduction in the availability of secure, easily accessible places to engage in physical recreation.

3. Lack of Sleep: Impairing Metabolism and Hormonal Balance

Getting enough sleep is crucial for both general wellbeing and keeping a healthy weight. Hormonal balance is upset by sleep loss, especially with regard to the levels of leptin and ghrelin, which control hunger and metabolism.

Leptin: An appetite suppressant and satiety signal produced by fat cells is called leptin. Lack of sleep lowers leptin levels, which increases desires and hunger, particularly for processed, high-calorie foods.

Ghrelin: The stomach secretes the hormone ghrelin, which increases hunger. Lack of sleep raises ghrelin levels, which intensifies appetite and makes it harder to restrict food consumption.

4. Emotional Eating: Using Food to Soothe Feelings

Emotional eating, or consuming food as a coping mechanism for stress, worry, or depression, can result in unhealthful eating patterns and weight gain. When people use food as a coping mechanism, they could overindulge or make poor eating decisions, which throws off their energy balance and increases the risk of obesity.

2. Psychological Aspects

1. Effect on Self-Regard

Obesity can create a dissonant thread during adolescence, a time of self-discovery and identity building, interfering with the rich experiences that should characterize this life-changing moment. Apart from the negative effects on physical health, teenage obesity has a major psychological influence, causing a cloud of self-doubt and low self-esteem that can significantly affect their general wellbeing.

People are particularly susceptible to peer acceptability and social perceptions during adolescence, making it a vulnerable time. Teens' self-esteem can be damaged by obesity, which is frequently stigmatized and linked to negative stereotypes. This can result in feelings of loneliness, anxiety, and sadness. These emotional loads can worsen poor eating patterns, starting a vicious cycle that is detrimental to their general wellbeing.

Research has consistently shown a strong correlation between teenage weight and low self-esteem. Teens who are obese frequently express feelings of being less attractive, less self-assured, and less accepted by their classmates. Their enjoyment of school life might be negatively impacted by this poor self-perception, which can also limit their engagement in extracurricular activities and hamper their social connections.

Beyond social connections, obesity has a psychological toll on teens' academic achievement and general mental health. Adolescents who are obese are more likely to experience anxiety, loneliness, and melancholy. These emotional weights may hinder their ability to focus, stay motivated, and perform well academically.

Additionally, the stigma attached to obesity can result in harassment and bullying, which exacerbates the psychological anguish that fat kids go through. They may limit their participation in sports, retreat from social interactions, and suffer feelings of shame and worthlessness as a result of their fear of social rejection and scorn.

Adolescent obesity can have long-term psychological effects that continue into adulthood. Anxiety, sadness, and low self-esteem can last into adulthood and have an impact on a person's relationships, professional choices, and general quality of life.

Teenage obesity has a negative impact on their mental and physical well-being in addition to their physical health. An all-encompassing strategy that supports mental health services, open communication, body positivity, healthy lifestyle choices, and self-acceptance is needed to properly address this problem. We can enhance the general well-being and opportunities for success in all aspects of life of obese teenagers by helping them to manage the psychological difficulties that come with gaining weight.

2. Patterns of Emotional Eating

People are particularly susceptible to peer acceptability and social perceptions during adolescence, making it a vulnerable time. Teens' self-esteem can be damaged by obesity, which is frequently stigmatized and linked to negative stereotypes. This can result in feelings of loneliness, anxiety, and sadness. These emotional loads can worsen poor eating patterns, starting a vicious cycle that is detrimental to their general wellbeing.

Among obese teenagers, emotional eating—eating to control or repress negative emotions—emerges as a common coping strategy. People seek brief release from emotional upheaval by turning to food for solace when they are experiencing stress, anxiety, sadness, loneliness, or boredom. Emotional eating patterns like these can be harmful to one's physical and mental well-being.

An emotional trigger, like a fight with a friend, stress from school, or loneliness, is often the first step in the cycle of emotional eating. Cravings for appetizing, frequently highly processed meals that bring comfort and satisfaction are triggered emotionally. People give in to their appetites and start eating excessively, consuming enormous amounts of food without thinking about how full they are or how hungry they are.

Uncontrolled eating is followed by a brief period of emotional distress reduction, which promotes peace and relaxation. But this fleeting reprieve is frequently followed by emotions of shame, remorse, and self-reproach, which exacerbates the underlying emotional pain. Because of this, people could feel stuck in a loop of emotional eating, constantly turning to food for solace and release, which would keep the pattern ongoing turning to food for comfort and relief.

Teens who are obese may develop emotional eating habits due to a number of circumstances, including:

Chronic Stress and Anxiety: Teenagers who experience chronic stress and anxiety are more likely to engage in emotional eating because of the ongoing pressures of schoolwork, extracurricular activities, and social expectations.

Low Self-Esteem: Because weight is stigmatized in society, obese teenagers frequently experience low self-esteem, which makes them turn to food for emotional support and comfort.

Learned Behaviors: Teenagers can imitate their parents' or other caregivers' emotional eating habits by using food as a coping mechanism for their own feelings.

Limited Coping Skills: Teens are more likely to turn to emotional eating because they may not have developed healthy coping

strategies for handling challenging emotions.
This is because of developmental reasons.

Beyond providing momentary solace from
emotional discomfort, emotional eating has
long-term negative effects on one's physical
and mental well-being.

Obesity and Weight Gain: Emotional eating
has been linked to obesity and weight gain,
which raises the risk of chronic conditions
like heart disease, type 2 diabetes, and
several malignancies.

Emotional Distress and Mood Swings: The
cycle of emotional eating can exacerbate
anxiety, melancholy, and guilt, which can
lead to a downward spiral of emotional
distress.

Reduced Self-Esteem: People who are unable
to regulate their emotional eating may have
a further decline in self-esteem as a result of
feeling helpless and unable to properly
control their emotions.

Social Isolation: Teens who binge eat emotionally may become socially isolated as a result of their withdrawal from relationships and activities because they feel ashamed and embarrassed.

Recall that ending the emotional eating cycle is a process rather than a destination. It calls for self-compassion, perseverance, and a readiness to make little adjustments. Teens who are obese can overcome emotional eating, create healthy coping skills, and take steps toward bettering their physical, mental, and social well-being with the correct help and techniques.

Chapter Two: Building Healthy Habits

It is crucial to take a realistic and nuanced approach while establishing healthy behaviors in obese kids. We promote sustainable techniques that go beyond weight control by highlighting small adjustments catered to the special requirements of puberty. This entails addressing overall well-being, which includes sleep patterns and stress management, in addition to nutritional instruction. It also entails developing healthy relationships with food and including pleasurable and sustainable physical activity. In order to build resilience, self-acceptance, and a basis for lifetime well-being, the objective is to enable teenagers to adopt better lives.

A. Gradual Transition: Adopting Small, Steady Steps

Adolescents who struggle with obesity encounter particular obstacles while trying to lead healthy lives. Cultivating healthy behaviors is essential to this shift, and it requires a sophisticated knowledge of the complexity involved. Adopting healthy behaviors in obese teenagers is a dynamic and intricate process that necessitates a strategy based on sustainability and small, gradual adjustments. We lay the groundwork for transformations that go beyond weight management and establish a basis for lifetime well-being by acknowledging the special problems of adolescence and designing interventions to fit the realities of teenage life. This method creates the foundation for a better and more rewarding future while also empowering teenagers to navigate their journey with self-acceptance and perseverance.

Setting off on a route towards healthy behaviors can be difficult, particularly for teenagers who are juggling the intricacies of their own preferences, social pressures, and body image. But encouraging durable lifestyle shifts necessitates a methodical approach that stresses baby, doable steps and puts long-term wellbeing ahead of short cures.

The human body is a complex system that changes with time. Although drastic lifestyle modifications may sound enticing for short-term gains, they might have unintended long-term consequences and frequently result in unsustainable practices. Rather, concentrating on small, regular steps can help create long-lasting habits.

Teenagers should be encouraged to think of small, doable adjustments they may make to their everyday activities. These adjustments could consist of:

Water or beverages without sugar can be used in place of sugary drinks.

Including extra fruits and vegetables in meals and snack foods

Substituting healthy snacks such as nuts, fruits, or yogurt for processed ones

During breaks or after school, going for quick walks or performing other mild exercise

These little actions might not seem like much, but they set the stage for long-term behavior modification and habit building.

There are obstacles to overcome on the path to good habits. Teens can experience disappointments, peer pressure, and moments of temptation. Urge them to embrace failures as teaching opportunities, refrain from self-criticism, and engage in self-compassion.

Recognize progress, celebrate little triumphs, and put more emphasis on long-term objectives than fleeting perfection. Teens should be reminded that they are not traveling alone and that friends, family, and medical professionals are here to support them.

Let's examine how important it is to help obese teens develop healthy habits, highlighting the need of small, long-lasting adjustments that take into account the reality of adolescence.

The understanding that developing healthy behaviors is a personalized process is at the core of this inquiry. Adolescents need a customized approach that takes into account their developmental stage, preferences, and specific circumstances as they navigate the turbulent waters of adolescence. Stressing progressive adjustments promotes a strategy that is both sustainable and aware of the need for adaptability, while also acknowledging the practical limitations and competing demands that teenagers must deal with.

For obese teenagers, incremental improvements are a more realistic and attainable course of action than complete overhauls. Adolescence is a time of many physical and emotional shifts, and enforcing drastic changes can be rather difficult. By promoting small, gradual changes to food habits, exercise routines, and general lifestyle choices, the emphasis is shifted from quick cures to long-lasting routines.

A key component of the worldview for developing healthful habits is sustainability. Instead than encouraging short-term remedies that might only produce fleeting effects, the focus is on developing long-term habits that become ingrained in a teen's everyday routine. Sustainable habits ensure that the adjustments achieved are not seen as transitory measures but rather as essential components of a lifelong journey towards health. They not only help with weight control but also enhance overall well-being.

Nutritional education that goes beyond calorie tracking is essential to this process. It entails imparting knowledge about portion management, balanced nutrition, and the nutritious properties of food. The emphasis is on developing a positive connection with food and encouraging an appreciation for its role in promoting health and vitality, as opposed to rigorous dieting. Teenagers are empowered to make sustainable eating choices when they are given the tools to prepare meals and make healthier food choices over time.

A similar philosophy of gradual inclusion is applied to physical activity, which is an essential part of a healthy lifestyle. Finding fun and sustainable kinds of exercise is important because teens may have different interests and differing levels of fitness. The idea is to integrate physical exercise into everyday life rather than forcing it into a schedule, whether that takes the form of individual workouts, organized sports, or leisure pursuits.

Furthermore, developing healthy habits involves more than just diet and exercise—it also involves managing stress, sleep patterns, and mental wellness. By attending to the holistic needs of teenagers, we may see the interdependence of several lifestyle factors and reaffirm that maintaining good health is a complex process.

Encouraging kids to develop healthy behaviors doesn't need making big or abrupt changes. It's about developing a lifetime of introspection, restraint, and environmentally friendly habits. Teens can take a stride toward holistic wellness and a better, happier future by accepting baby steps, emphasizing long-term well-being, and cultivating self-compassion.

1.Nutritional Guidance

The goal of nutritional counseling for obese teenagers is to encourage a well-balanced diet that includes whole grains, fruits, vegetables, lean meats, and healthy fats. Portion control, calorie monitoring, and the significance of staying hydrated are stressed. Fostering good eating habits in obese teenagers requires a comprehensive and long-lasting strategy that includes tailoring recommendations to individual preferences, educating teens about nutritional labels, and seeking professional help.

i. Promoting Health with Suggestions for a Balanced Diet

An all-encompassing and customized strategy is necessary to address the dietary demands of obese teenagers. The majority of this conversation centers on offering suggestions for a balanced diet, acknowledging the significance of sustenance, sustainability, and personal preferences in fostering long-term health.

Encouraging teens with obesity to follow balanced diet recommendations include educating them about nutrition, encouraging variety, and taking into account their personal tastes. In addition to helping with weight management, this all-encompassing strategy establishes the groundwork for wholesome eating practices that last a lifetime, giving them the confidence and knowledge to make informed nutritional decisions.

1. Having an Understanding of a Balanced Diet: A balanced diet consists of a range of foods high in nutrients that supply vital macronutrients, vitamins, and minerals. Essential elements comprise fruits, vegetables, whole grains, lean meats, and healthy fats, providing a variety of nutrients essential for development and growth.

2. Calorie Awareness and Portion Control: Portion control is essential for assisting youngsters in controlling their calorie consumption without turning to restrictive diets. Raising students' understanding of food portions and nutritional values allows to make healthier choices.

3. Making Fruits and Vegetables a Priority: Promoting a diverse and colorful diet of fruits and vegetables guarantees a wealth of antioxidants, vitamins, and minerals. Stressing these elements naturally reduces calorie consumption while laying the groundwork for general wellness.

4. Whole Grains for Long-Term Energy Release: Complex carbs included in whole grains like brown rice, quinoa, and whole wheat allow for long-term energy release. They also provide fiber, which helps with digestion and encourages fullness.

5. Lean Proteins for Muscle Health: Eating foods high in lean protein, such as fish, chicken, lentils, and tofu, helps to maintain and build muscle. Because they increase sensations of fullness, proteins help prevent overindulging in calories.

6. Moderate Intake of Healthy Fats: Consuming almonds, avocados, and olive oil are good sources of healthy fats that are essential for brain health and general wellbeing. These foods can be high in calories, thus moderation is essential. This highlights the significance of balance.

7. Hydration as a Cornerstone: Drinking enough water is essential for good health and can help control weight by making you feel fuller. Water consumption should be

prioritised above sugary drinks in order to promote hydration without consuming extra calories.

8. Tailoring Recommendations to Individual interests: It's important to acknowledge that every adolescent has different interests and tastes. Personalized dietary advice based on personal preferences enhances the chances of long-term compliance with a well-rounded diet.

9. Nutritional Label Education: Giving teenagers the skills to decipher nutritional labels gives them the confidence to choose foods based on their own knowledge. Teenagers are more equipped to negotiate the complexity of packaged goods when they are aware of concepts like portion size, daily values, and ingredient lists.

10. Seeking Professional Advice: Consulting with nutritionists or dietitians in cases of obesity guarantees individualized and scientifically supported dietary advice. A complete approach to dietary adjustments is

ensured by the assistance of a professional in addressing certain health concerns.

3. Nutritional Counseling for Obesity-Stricken Teens

Obesity can become a major issue in the complex structure of adolescence, affecting not just physical health but also mental and social well-being. In order to solve this problem, nutritional education is essential since it gives teenagers the power to choose foods wisely and create a balanced diet that promotes their general health and wellbeing.

Important Guidelines for a Balanced Diet

Teens who are obese and on a balanced diet should follow these important guidelines:

Enough Calorie Consumption: It is important to take into account several parameters, including age, gender, height, activity level, and current weight status, when determining the optimum calorie intake for each individual. A medical expert can offer tailored advice on caloric consumption objectives.

Encourage a diet that is varied and full of a range of nutrient-dense foods, such as fruits, vegetables, whole grains, and lean protein sources. Essential vitamins, minerals, and fiber from these foods promote general health and wellbeing.

Processed Foods: Reduce your intake of processed meals, sugar-filled beverages, and harmful fats. These meals raise the risk of developing chronic diseases and causing weight gain since they are frequently heavy in calories, sugar, bad fats, and sodium.

Control of Portion: To guarantee a balanced nutrient intake and avoid overindulging, practice mindful eating and portion control. When eating, use smaller dishes, portion out snacks, and keep your eyes off of other things.

Regular Meal routine: To avoid overindulging in food or unhealthy snacking, stick to a regular meal routine. Throughout the day, consume two to three snacks in addition to three big meals.

Hydration: To promote general health and avoid dehydration, encourage a sufficient consumption of water throughout the day. In addition to aiding in fullness, water helps lessen cravings for sugary beverages.

In order to provide further context for the ideas behind a balanced diet, the following is a thorough analysis of the food suggestions for obese teenagers:

Produce and Fruits: Try to consume five or more servings of fruits and vegetables each day. To increase nutrient intake, incorporate a range of hues and varieties.

Whole Grains: Whenever feasible, opt for whole grains rather than refined ones. Fiber, vitamins, and minerals included in whole grains help with blood sugar regulation, digestion, and overall health.

Lean Protein Sources: Take into account a range of lean protein sources, including low-fat dairy products, fish, chicken, beans, and lentils. Protein aids in tissue healing, muscle growth, and satiety.

Healthy Fats: Include fats that are good for you, such as those found in olive oil, avocados, nuts, and seeds. These fats boost heart health and offer vital nutrients.

Restricted Sugary Drinks: Reduce your intake of sugary beverages such as juices, sodas, and coffee drinks that have been sweetened. These beverages lead to tooth decay and weight gain by offering empty calories.

Decreased Processed Foods: Try consuming fewer processed foods, like sugary cereals, fast meals, and packaged snacks. These foods frequently contain large amounts of sodium, bad fats, and calories.

Portion control and Mindful Eating: Engage in mindful eating by savoring food, being aware of your hunger cues, and slowing down mealtimes.

Regular Meal routine: To avoid overindulging in food or unhealthy snacking, stick to a regular meal routine. Throughout the day, consume two to three snacks in addition to three big meals.

Teens who are obese can make educated food choices, create healthy eating habits, and promote their general well-being by following these balanced diet guidelines.

 Teenage obesity is caused by a number of variables, including environmental factors, lifestyle choices, and heredity. Portion control is an important but frequently ignored element.

Portion control is eating the appropriate amount of food for your needs. This entails eating till you are satisfied but not overfull. It also means not overindulging in food, no matter how good or easy to get it may be.

It becomes clear that portion management is essential to understanding and treating teen obesity. Rapid growth and development during adolescence is accompanied by a greater degree of independence when it comes to eating. Portion management is crucial to understanding teenage obesity because it's a useful and efficient way to control caloric intake. Teens can form healthy habits that promote their general well-being and play a major role in preventing and managing obesity-related issues by being taught about proper portion sizes.

Teens' bodies are continually changing during a critical period in their development. They must avoid overeating, which can result in weight gain and other health issues, but they must also consume enough calories to support their growth and activity.

Teens can take charge of their health and lower their risk of obesity and other linked health issues by practicing portion control. It's critical to keep in mind that maintaining portion control is only one aspect of a healthy lifestyle. Along with these healthy habits, teens should prioritize eating a balanced diet, exercising frequently, and making other wise decisions.

The following are some of the main arguments in favor of portion restriction as a strategy for treating teen obesity:

lowers consumption of calories: Eating less calories naturally results in smaller portions, which can support good weight maintenance.

Enhances the quality of your diet: By emphasizing smaller quantities, you are more likely to select nutrient-dense foods that will make you feel content and full.

Encourages the development of lifelong healthy eating habits: Teaching teens portion management at a young age can help them form lifelong healthy eating habits.

Lowers risk of chronic diseases: Type 2 diabetes, heart disease, and several types of cancer are just a few of the chronic diseases for which obesity is a significant risk factor. Teenagers can lower their lifetime risk of acquiring these diseases by exercising portion control.

Enhances self-esteem: Teens' confidence and self-esteem can be enhanced by maintaining a healthy weight.

1. Knowledge of Calorie:.Portion control raises teenagers' knowledge of calories and helps them comprehend how much energy is in their food. Being aware of portion sizes helps you make wise decisions and avoid consuming too many calories, which can lead to weight gain.

2. Preventing Overeating: Adolescents who are obese may struggle with emotional eating or ingesting more food than their bodies need. Controlling portion sizes helps avoid overindulging, promotes better eating

habits, and lowers the chance of gaining too much weight.

3. Balanced Nutrient Intake: Limiting portion sizes promotes a more even nutrient distribution. A varied and nutrient-rich diet is encouraged by making sure that the right amounts of fruits, vegetables, proteins, and grains are consumed, which supports general health.

4. Habit Formation: Portion control education creates enduring behaviors that support healthy weight management. Recognizing proper portion sizes in adolescents increases the likelihood that they will carry this information into adulthood and avoid obesity-related issues.

5. Avoiding Restrictive Diets: Portion control helps teens avoid the drawbacks of restrictive diets, which they might not be able to stick to. It encourages eating in a balanced way, making it possible to enjoy a range of foods without going without.

6. Preventing Mindless Eating: During meals, teenagers are frequently distracted by electronics or hectic schedules, which can result in mindless eating. Portion control promotes conscious eating and strengthens the link between hunger signals and food intake.

7. Tailored Approach: Teenagers have different nutritional demands depending on their metabolism, degree of exercise, and development rate. Portion control acknowledges that there is no one-size-fits-all method for managing obesity and permits a customized approach.

8. Long-Term Health Impact: Portion management helps maintain long-term health by halting the onset or aggravation of diseases linked to obesity, such as type 2 diabetes and heart problems. Adolescent habits lower the risk of chronic diseases in adulthood and lay the groundwork for healthier living.

Advice on portion control for teenagers:

Make use of tiny dishes and plates: You can fool your brain into thinking that you can eat less food by doing this.

Examine the labeling on food: Be mindful of portion sizes and ensure that you are not consuming more than is advised.

Consume food slowly and thoroughly chew it: You are less prone to overeat since this allows your brain time to recognize when you are satisfied.

Steer clear of distractions when eating: You're more likely to eat mindlessly and consume more food than you need when you're preoccupied with other activities, like watching TV or using your phone.

Make a plan for your meals and snacks to help you stay away from bad options and ensure that you consume a balanced diet all day long.

Engage in regular exercise: Exercise aids in calorie burning and weight maintenance.

Chapter Three: Nurturing Positive Body Image for Teens with Obesity: Fostering Self-Acceptance and Resilience

Developing a healthy body image is essential to overall wellbeing in the setting of teen obesity. Adolescence, a time of physical transitions and social demands, can pose particular difficulties for adolescents who are obese.

Adolescents with obesity require complex tactics that go beyond physical appearance to foster a positive body image. Teenagers may establish a better relationship with their bodies and lay the foundation for a positive self-image and lifetime well-being by encouraging self-acceptance, questioning social standards, and building resilience.

Let's examine the value of developing a positive body image, self-acceptance techniques, and perseverance in overcoming the challenges associated with body perception.

1. Redefining Beauty Standards: It's critical to inspire teenagers to reevaluate and challenge conventional notions of beauty. A sense of tolerance is fostered by highlighting diversity and questioning restrictive ideas, which teaches youth that beauty can take many forms.

2. Open Communication: It is essential to create channels of communication that are both judgment-free and open at home and in educational environments. Teens should be free to open up about their experiences, worries, and sentiments around body image without worrying about being judged.

3. Prioritizing Health Over attractiveness: Putting health above attractiveness encourages a more optimistic outlook. Teens are more likely to believe that health is a holistic concept that extends beyond outward appearances if they are encouraged to participate in activities that enhance their general well-being.

4. Media literacy instruction: Teaching teenagers media literacy skills enables them to evaluate how bodies are portrayed in the media. Teens who are aware of how the media shapes body ideals are more equipped to evaluate these messages and make wise decisions.

5. Encouraging Self-Compassion: Teaching teenagers to accept their flaws and treat themselves with kindness is a key component in encouraging self-compassion. Fostering a self-love and self-awareness mindset helps combat negative self-talk and advances a positive self-image.

6. Recognizing and Challenging Negative attitudes: It's critical to help kids identify and confront negative attitudes they may have about their bodies. To develop a more optimistic outlook and modify negative thought patterns, cognitive-behavioral techniques might be utilized.

7. Celebrating Non-Physical Attributes: Diversifying sources of self-worth can be achieved by acknowledging and appreciating non-physical traits like kindness, intelligence, and resilience. Teens are encouraged by this method to value who they are outside of their appearance.

8. Promoting Positive Affirmations: Using affirmations that are specific to a person's accomplishments and strengths helps to strengthen a positive self-perception. Maintaining a regular affirmation practice helps lay the groundwork for confidence and self-worth.

9. Including Support Networks: Including mentors, family members, and friends who are encouraging builds a network of support. Adolescents who have a robust support network find it easier to overcome obstacles and to embrace messages about their bodies.

10. Developing Resilience: For teenagers dealing with social pressures over their weight, developing resilience is essential. Stressing that obstacles are a natural part of life and can present chances for development helps people become resilient and overcome hardship.

For teenagers who are battling obesity, the following are some essential tactics to foster a positive self-perception:

1. Act as an Example: Refrain from condemning your own body and instead practice self-compassion. Teens are quick to pick up on and internalize the language we use about ourselves. Pay attention to what you say and do, and show that you embrace and value your physical appearance.

Put your body's skills and functions first rather than merely its size or shape when discussing your health and ability. This teaches teenagers that their bodies are useful tools for resilience, strength, and mobility.

2. Contest Images in the Media: Talk about the inaccurate depictions of beauty in the media: Discuss how fabricated improvements, filters, and editing are used to produce unattainable body standards. Teens can use this to sharpen their critical thinking abilities and learn the difference between real bodies and Photoshopped ones.

Introduce them to a range of body types: Urge kids to watch and read media that highlights the variety of people's bodies, sizes, and ethnicities on social media. They learn from this that beauty can take many different forms.

3. Foster Self-Acceptance: Promote awareness and assist teenagers in realizing their abilities and qualities that go beyond outward appearances. This highlights their own attributes and potential, fostering self-worth and confidence.

Encourage teenagers to embrace body neutrality by teaching them to see their bodies as tools for living, not as things to be critiqued. This encourages people to stop worrying so much about how they look and instead value their bodies for what they can do.

4. Promote Good Relationships: Promote wholesome friendships: Provide kids with a helpful and welcoming peer group to help them develop a positive body image and a love for themselves.

Establish a comfortable environment for candid communication by promoting frank discussions regarding self-esteem and body image. Actively listen and provide assistance without passing judgment.

5. Honor individuality: Promote originality and self-expression in teenagers by assisting them in discovering methods to express themselves via their choices of attire, pastimes, and personal flair. This fosters a feeling of confidence in their individuality and self-ownership.

Concentrate on your own objectives: Encourage teenagers to create goals for their whole wellbeing and health rather than simply their looks. This encourages children to adopt healthy habits for internal rather than external reasons.

Recall that developing a good body image is a process rather than a final goal. We can assist teenagers in developing a positive relationship with their bodies and provide them the tools they need to take care of their wellbeing by being kind, encouraging, and patient with them.

1. Concentrating on General Health and Welfare

Strictly concentrating on weight loss can be detrimental to kids who are obese and result in a bad body image. Putting a strong emphasis on general health and wellbeing turns out to be an effective tactic for fostering a positive body image among obese teenagers. Teens may cultivate a resilient mindset, value themselves above and beyond societal norms, and start down the path to a healthy and affirming connection with their bodies by changing the narrative to promote holistic wellbeing. This method can be more successful in promoting good body image and long-lasting behavior change, in addition to supporting immediate well-being and laying the groundwork for a lifetime enjoyment of health in all its dimensions.

How to do it is as follows:

1. Take Weight Loss Out of the Picture: Give up on tight diets and overexertion in the gym. These behaviors have the potential to be detrimental and raise low self-esteem.

Pay attention to good habits for their own sakc. Encourage teenagers to emphasize getting enough sleep and managing their stress, eat healthily, and participate in physical activity they like.

Rejoice in non-scale accomplishments. Acknowledge and value gains in general health, mood, and energy levels in addition to weight fluctuations.

2. Encourage Body Appreciation: Assist teenagers in recognizing and appreciating the assets and qualities of their bodies. Consider their physical capabilities rather than just their appearance.

Promote self-care routines. Encourage them to engage in healthy body-mind exercises like yoga, meditation, and massage.

Speak in a body-positive manner. Refrain from criticizing someone's size, weight, or looks. Instead, emphasize language that is neutral or affirming.

3. Promote Confidence and Self-Esteem: Assist teenagers in realizing their abilities and qualities that go beyond outward appearances. Motivate them to pursue their passions and hone their special skills.

Stop talking to yourself negatively. Assist teenagers in recognizing and combating self-defeating ideas about their appearance.

Honor achievements and triumphs. To help kids develop self-worth and confidence, encourage them to set reasonable goals and recognize their accomplishments.

4. Seek Professional Assistance if Needed: Take into Account Getting Professional Assistance from a Licensed Dietician or Therapist. They can offer tailored advice and assistance to teenagers who are having issues with their bodies or their diet.

5. Encouraging Healthy Habits: A constructive emphasis is placed on encouraging healthy habits, such as a balanced diet and regular exercise. Stressing the value of being strong, resilient, and full of energy helps people feel well-being that goes beyond controlling their weight.

6. Goal Setting Beyond Appearance: It's critical to expand goal-setting conversations

to include a variety of accomplishments that go beyond outward appearance. Teens are reinforced in their worth beyond the opinions of others when they are encouraged to set goals pertaining to their academic performance, personal development, and community service.

7. Mindful Eating Practices: Developing conscious and constructive relationships with food is facilitated by implementing mindful eating practices. A healthier mentality is facilitated by concentrating on the sensory experience of eating, identifying signs of hunger and fullness, and appreciating the nutritional qualities of food.

8. Positive Reinforcement for Healthful Choices: Providing encouragement for healthful decisions strengthens a favorable link with wellbeing, regardless of weight-related consequences. Acknowledging the efforts made to develop better behaviors helps one feel more accomplished and valuable.

9. Inclusive Physical Activities: Promoting inclusive physical activities that put more emphasis on having fun than losing weight helps people develop a good rapport with exercise. A sensation of achievement and physical empowerment are enhanced by engaging in activities that highlight movement and skill development.

10. The promotion of body positivity and representation in educational materials and media is vital. A more accepting and encouraging atmosphere for obese teenagers is created when different body shapes are acknowledged and embraced.

It is possible to establish a conducive atmosphere that promotes positive body image and gives them the confidence to make healthy decisions for themselves by emphasizing overall health and wellbeing. For obese teenagers, a healthy and fulfilling life can be encouraged by this all-encompassing approach that can result in long-lasting behavioral improvements.

2. Encouraging Self-Acceptance and Steering Clear of Negative Remarks

Promoting self-acceptance and reducing critical remarks are essential components in helping obese teenagers develop a healthy body image. In the process of helping obese kids develop a healthy body image, encouraging self-acceptance and reducing hurtful remarks are essential. This approach attempts to create an atmosphere that encourages self-love and resilience while acknowledging the importance of both external factors and one's own self-perception on one's body image.

One effective tactic for fostering a positive body image in obese teenagers is encouraging self-acceptance and avoiding negative comments. Teens can create a resilient attitude that lays the groundwork for a good and affirming connection with their bodies by cultivating an environment that stresses self-worth beyond looks, providing tools to handle cultural pressures, and encouraging open communication. This method helps youth deal with the challenges of body image throughout their lifetimes, in addition to supporting their immediate well-being.

Here are a few particular tactics to help you accomplish this:

1. Develop Acceptance: Promote kindness and self-compassion. Assist teenagers in appreciating and recognizing their own traits, as well as their worth beyond outward appearances.

Stop talking to yourself negatively. Recognize and swap out negative self-talk about their bodies for empowering statements and self-affirmations.

Pay attention to internal attributes. Empathy is strengthened when the focus is shifted from outward appearance to within attributes. Promoting kids' self-awareness and appreciation of their skills, generosity, and intelligence helps them develop a more complete sense of who they are.

It is essential to create an atmosphere that welcomes diversity and values individual differences. Creating an accepting culture at home, in the classroom, and among peers helps to create a welcoming environment.

2. Minimize Negativity Exposure:

Determine the negative triggers. Assist teenagers in recognizing the individuals, circumstances, or media that exacerbate bad body image and self-esteem.

Create coping skills. Give teenagers the skills they need to control their emotions and react constructively to criticism.

Encourage responsible use of social media. Advise teenagers to watch videos and follow accounts that promote self-acceptance and body positivity.

Encourage responsible use of social media. Advise teenagers to watch videos and follow accounts that promote self-acceptance and body positivity.

Teaching teenagers about the representation of bodies in the media and its influences aids in the development of a critical mindset. Examining and challenging the exaggerated ideals of beauty propagated by the media cultivates resistance to harmful social messages.

3. Respond to Critical Remarks: Improve Your Communication Abilities. Teach teenagers how to stand up for themselves and react politely to criticism of their appearance.

Ask for help from responsible adults. Teens should be encouraged to confide in dependable adults such as mentors, parents, or teachers.

Put your attention toward developing resilience. Assist teenagers in learning how to overcome adversity and preserve their self-confidence.

Teens will feel supported if a safe environment is established where they can talk freely about hurtful remarks.

4. Use neutral language and good body language to encourage body-positive communication. Steer clear of disparaging remarks about size, weight, or looks.

Highlight each person's accomplishments and strengths. Honor non-scale successes as well as each teen's distinct skills and abilities.

Stress the value of being healthy and happy. Talk about the relationship between good habits and general well-being.

5. Establish a Supportive Environment: Set an example of acceptance of who you are. Avoid making disparaging remarks about your appearance and instead show that you value and appreciate your own body.

Encourage direct and sincere communication. Encourage teenagers to openly express their thoughts and worries about their bodies without fear of rejection.

Honor uniqueness and diversity. Encourage the creation of a culture that respects and honors people of all ages, sizes, and races.

3. Highlighting Success and Promoting Development

For obese teenagers, acknowledging accomplishments and promoting advancement are essential components of a healthy body image. We can encourage people to keep going on their path to health and well-being by highlighting their accomplishments.

Fostering a positive body image in obese kids can be accomplished through empowering and dynamically celebrating progress and accomplishments. With this strategy, kids are given the tools to see their value beyond outward appearances by emphasizing individual successes, acknowledging personal growth, and creating a supportive environment. In addition to improving their well-being right away, it establishes the groundwork for a strong and healthy relationship with their bodies that will last a lifetime.

Here are some particular tactics to put this into practice:

1. Celebrate and Acknowledge Non-Scale Victories:

Pay attention to gains in mood, energy, and general health. Acknowledge and commemorate these beneficial developments as indicators of advancement.

Appreciate the rise in physical exercise. Recognize their attempts to move their bodies in ways they enjoy, whether it's taking up a new activity, going on more walks, or dancing in their room.

Draw attention to the development of healthy behaviors. Acknowledge and encourage them for making healthy food choices and self-care routines a part of their everyday lives.

2. Establish Individualized and Realistic Goals: Assist teenagers in establishing attainable and realistic goals. These objectives ought to be SMART—specific, measurable, achievable, relevant, and time-bound.

Prioritize your own objectives over those of others. Teens should be encouraged to set meaningful objectives for themselves and to recognize and appreciate their accomplishments in light of their unique beginnings.

Appreciate your little progress along the way. Acknowledge and celebrate each step they take to reach their objectives to help them feel motivated and accomplished.

Teens who are encouraged to set reasonable and doable goals feel more empowered and have a sense of autonomy. Progress is valued and a positive self-perception is reinforced by little, incremental victories.

3. Make Use of Positive Reinforcement: Give more attention to praising effort and advancement than size or looks. Teens benefit from this by internalizing the worth of their work and staying motivated.

Give sincere, targeted compliments. Give them particular appreciation for their actions, accomplishments, or character traits rather than just platitudes.

Put techniques for positive reinforcement to use. To sustain their enthusiasm and motivate them to keep going, think about offering incentives or awards.

4. Encourage a Growth Mindset: Assist teenagers in viewing obstacles and failures as chances to improve. Urge them to view errors as opportunities for growth rather than as signs of failure.

Put your attention on perseverance and effort. Instill in them the value of perseverance and hard work in accomplishing their objectives.

Honor tenacity and fortitude. Recognize their capacity to overcome obstacles and recover from failures.

5. Encourage Self-efficacy: Assist teenagers in forging a solid belief in their own capacity to succeed. To help them become more confident, encourage them to list their advantages and prior accomplishments.

Give people the chance to hone their skills and become proficient. Provide assistance and direction as they pick up new abilities and form wholesome routines.

Give them the freedom to decide for themselves. Promote a sense of control and independence in them by encouraging them to take charge of their health and well-being.

6. Acknowledging Non-Physical Achievements: It is important to refocus attention from physical appearance to non-physical achievements. Honoring achievements in the classroom, personal development, and constructive contributions strengthens a sense of accomplishment on all fronts.

7. Stressing inner value: Stressing an individual's inherent worth above and beyond outward indicators promotes self-esteem. Promoting a healthy self-image in teenagers involves helping them to see their contributions and special talents.

8. Establishing a Positive Feedback Loop: A motivating environment can be created by establishing a positive feedback loop through the recognition of accomplishments. Acknowledging endeavors and advancements, irrespective of magnitude, strengthens a feeling of success.

9. Fostering Self-Reflection: Self-reflection enables teenagers to recognize their own development. Positive body image is enhanced by helping them to recognize and appreciate the strides they have made toward health and wellbeing.

10. Offering concrete incentives: Positive behavior is reinforced when efforts and accomplishments are met with concrete incentives. These incentives don't have to do with weight; they might be linked to positive behaviors, self-care, or individual achievements.

11. Celebrating Personal progress: Highlighting achievements that show tenacity, personal progress, and conquering obstacles helps to strengthen a positive self-narrative. A healthy way of thinking is to acknowledge the journey instead of obsessing over the end point.

12. Creating a friendly Environment: A friendly atmosphere that values accomplishments encourages a feeling of

community. Promoting participation from mentors, family, and friends in success celebrations helps create a happy environment.

13. Including Mindfulness Activities: Including mindfulness activities, such self-affirmation and gratitude exercises, helps youth concentrate on their positive traits. These behaviors support a healthy body image and foster a more upbeat outlook.

14. Strengthening Intrinsic Motivation: Stressing the idea that achievements stem from a person's own fulfillment rather than approval from others helps people develop a long-lasting good self-perception. Teens with resilient and optimistic mindsets are fostered when they are encouraged to find joy and fulfillment in their journey.

Chapter Four: Integrating Physical Activity in Teen Obesity

For the purpose of controlling teen obesity and advancing general health and wellbeing, physical activity is essential. Nonetheless, incorporating physical exercise into the lives of obese teenagers necessitates thoughtful planning and approaches that take into account their capabilities, interests, and needs. Here are some important tactics and advantages to think about:

Techniques:

1. Discovering Pleasurable Pastimes:

Assist teenagers in discovering activities that they truly love, rather than just what they consider to be "exercise." Sports, dancing, swimming, hiking, and other activities that get kids moving and having fun can all fall under this category.

Give them a range of options to consider. Teens should be encouraged to try a variety of activities to see what interests and stimulates them.

Pay attention to the social aspects of exercise. To make exercising more enjoyable and social, play team sports, sign up for group fitness courses, or work out with pals.

Creating engaging activities with social components improves motivation. Team sports, fitness competitions, and group sessions foster a sense of camaraderie and elevate physical activity to a pleasurable experience.

2. Creating Accessibility for Physical Activity:

Eliminate obstacles to involvement. Take into account any expenses, travel, or scheduling conflicts that would keep them from participating in regular physical activity.

Provide a range of possibilities. Provide options that suit a range of requirements and preferences by including varied exercise lengths, intensities, and locations.

Encourage movement all through the day. Urge teenagers to include physical activity in their everyday schedules by encouraging them to walk during breaks or use the stairs rather than the elevator.

Promoting commuting by bicycle or walking, when possible, integrates physical exercise into everyday schedules. In addition to improving health, active transportation incorporates movement throughout daily life.

3. Creating Practical Objectives:

As you make progress, progressively increase the duration and intensity of your goals from tiny, manageable beginnings. This fosters a feeling of success and helps keep discouragement at bay.

Prioritize progress over perfection. No matter how tiny the increase in physical activity may seem, it should be celebrated.

Based on your skills and degree of fitness, set personal objectives. Advise them to concentrate on their own journey and refrain from comparing their progress to others'.

Setting attainable and realistic workout objectives makes you feel accomplished. Honouring accomplishments in the areas of strength, endurance, and skill development promotes positive behaviour.

4. Creating a Supportive Network: Promote joining sports teams or group fitness classes. This offers social support, accountability, and a feeling of community.

Determine virtuous role models. Teens should be surrounded by people who value physical activity and promote healthy lifestyle choices.

Offer your family and friends' encouragement and support. As they progress, acknowledge their accomplishments and give them encouragement.

Promoting physical activity within the family creates a supportive atmosphere. Family bonding is strengthened and fitness is promoted by engaging in sports, hiking, or other outdoor activities.

5. Customised Approach: Customising physical activity regimens to meet each person's needs and preferences guarantees participation. Diverse interests are catered to by providing a range of possibilities, including team sports, solitary pastimes, and recreational pursuits.

6. Gradual Progression: Adolescents can develop endurance by gradually increasing the intensity and duration of their workouts. It is less likely to become discouraged and to sustain an injury if you begin with activities that are doable and then progressively increase in intensity.

7. Using Technology: Adding interactive games, virtual classes, or fitness apps to actual exercise increases its appeal. Teens with tech-savvy tastes can find diversity and attraction in technology.

Benefits:

1. Better Physical Health: Lower chance of obesity-related illnesses such heart disease, type 2 diabetes, and specific cancers.

-improved endurance, flexibility, and strength.

-increased vitality and better quality of sleep.

-enhanced capacity of the immunological system.

2. Improved Mental Health: Diminished signs of depression and anxiety.

-enhanced confidence and sense of self-worth.

-happier and more content all around.

-decreased stress and enhanced coping skills.

Engaging in physical activity can improve mental health by lowering stress and anxiety. Exercise causes endorphins to be released, which enhances pleasure and wellbeing.

3. Development of Healthful Habits: Encourages the adoption of a lifelong healthy lifestyle.

-promotes beneficial behaviors and the consumption of healthful foods.

-gives a way to unwind and relieve tension.

-increases drive and self-control.

The basis for lifetime fitness is laid during youth by forming a habit of frequent physical activity. Active teenagers are more likely to maintain these practices throughout adulthood.

4. Creating Social Connections: Offers chances for communication and companionship.

-encourages a feeling of community and belonging.

-enhances communication and social skills.

-promotes cooperation and teamwork.

Engaging in collective endeavors promotes interpersonal communication and a feeling of inclusion. Emotional health is enhanced by positive social interactions.

5. Weight Management: Maintaining a healthy weight and avoiding obesity require regular physical activity. It promotes a healthy metabolism and aids in the burning of calories.

6. Cardiovascular Health: Cardiovascular health is improved by aerobic exercise, which lowers the risk of heart-related problems. Heart health and circulation are linked to general well-being.

7. Better Body Image: Regular exercise is associated with better body image and

self-esteem. Reaching fitness objectives increases confidence and one's sense of accomplishment.

8. Improved Academic Performance: Research indicates that physical exercise and academic achievement are positively correlated. Exercise enhances focus, cognitive function, and general academic performance.

1. Identifying Enjoyable Physical Activities: A Key to Integrating Activity in Teen Obesity Management

Promoting regular physical activity among obese teenagers is essential for their overall health and wellbeing. This method acknowledges the value of making exercise enjoyable and motivating, as it improves general wellbeing in addition to helping people manage their weight.

But the conventional method of pressuring children into particular sports or workout regimens frequently results in resistance and, eventually, disengagement. Finding engaging physical activities that they truly connect with is essential to success.

Teens battling obesity can effectively integrate exercise into their life by identifying and fostering fun physical activities. By emphasizing the value of fun, using cooperative decision-making, and fostering a supportive atmosphere, we enable teenagers to view physical activity as a healthy and long-lasting part of their lives. This method not only helps control weight but also creates the groundwork for a lifetime of pleasurable and healthful exercise routines.

The following techniques can assist teenagers in finding and embracing hobbies they will love:

Examine a Variety of Options:

Transcend the conventional exercise regimen. Provide a variety of activities, such as athletics, dance, yoga, martial arts, sports, swimming, biking, hiking, rock climbing, and even movement-based video games.

Think about personal preferences. Encourage teenagers to choose their hobbies, whether they are team sports, solitary endeavors, outdoor, or indoor pastimes.

This approach lays the foundation for a lifetime of enjoyable and beneficial exercise routines in addition to aiding with weight control.

Teens looking to discover and embrace interests they will love can benefit from the following strategies:

Consider a Range of Choices:

Go beyond the traditional workout plan. Offer a range of activities, including swimming, biking, hiking, rock climbing, dance, yoga, martial arts, athletics, and even electronic games that require mobility.

Consider your own tastes. Teens should be encouraged to select their own hobbies, whether they be solo pursuits, team sports, or indoor or outdoor activities.

Arrange fun, active get-togethers with loved ones. Take group activities like biking, hiking, or sports to foster camaraderie and social connection.

3. Dismantle obstacles and Promote Experimentation:

Take care of any practical issues. Take into account any time, money, or transportation restrictions that might prevent participation.

Provide inexpensive or free options. Investigate parks, community centers, and internet resources that offer inexpensive or free access to a range of activities.

Promote experimenting with new things. Give teenagers the chance to try out several things without having to commit, so they can find their hidden interests and talents.

Teens should be encouraged to try a variety of activities to find what they prefer. Stress that it's common to try out a variety of workouts before settling on the ones that you enjoy the most.

4. Collaborate with Peers and Role Models:

Put teenagers in touch with wholesome role models who partake in enjoyable physical activities. Observing people enjoying themselves while exercising can be inspiring.

Encourage friends or peers with comparable interests to participate. This fosters a positive atmosphere and raises the possibility of ongoing participation.

Include gamification and technology. Examine wearable technology, interactive games, and fitness apps that can enhance the enjoyment and engagement of physical exercise.

5. Honor Progress and Achievements: Honor every increase in physical activity, no matter how long or how hard it lasts. This

encourages teenagers to keep working hard and develop a regular physical lifestyle.

Consider their own path and development rather than making comparisons with others. This gives them confidence in themselves and gives them the ability to set realistic goals.

Give them modest tokens of gratitude or enjoyable experiences in exchange for their efforts. This keeps people motivated by providing positive reinforcement.

6. Including Interests: Connect physical activity to current interests or hobbies. Teens who like dancing, for instance, can benefit from dance-based lessons or workouts.

7. Adaptable and Flexible Methods: Acknowledge that tastes can shift and that adaptability is essential. Sustaining engagement requires adaptability and a willingness to try out novel experiences.

8. Using Technology: Use technology to add interest to your operations. The use of apps,

online courses, or virtual experiences can make working out more engaging and entertaining.

9. Setting Reasonable Expectations: Recognize that development can take some time and set reasonable expectations. Stress the process of finding fun activities to include in your overall exercise regimen.

Remember, the goal is not to force teens into specific activities, but to empower them to explore and discover what they truly enjoy. We can assist overweight teenagers in incorporating physical activity into their lives by creating a joyful and upbeat atmosphere, promoting social contact, and recognizing their accomplishments.

Importance of Enjoyable Physical Activities

1. Sustainable Engagement: Long-term retention of enjoyable activities is higher. When their workout regimen is enjoyable and fits with their interests, teens are more likely to stick with it.

2. Positive Associations with Exercise: Teenagers are more likely to associate exercise positively when they find physical activity enjoyable. This optimistic outlook lowers the likelihood that exercise will be seen as a chore and fosters a healthy relationship with fitness.

3. Intrinsic Motivation: Pleasurable activities promote intrinsic motivation, in which the enjoyment of the action acts as a catalyst. Sustained engagement and a greater chance of forming a lifelong habit of physical activity are associated with intrinsic motivation.

4. Emotional Well-Being: Taking part in joyful activities enhances emotional well-being. When exercise is fun, it can improve mental health and lower stress, which can elevate mood.

5. Variety and Exploration: Helping teenagers find fun things to do inspires them to look into a range of possibilities. Teens who are exposed to a variety of exercise styles are better able to find what works for

them, which encourages a varied and comprehensive approach to fitness.

6. Confidence Building: Confidence is bolstered by accomplishment and enjoyment in physical activity. Good experiences boost self-esteem and self-efficacy by creating a sense of accomplishment.

7. Social Connection: Social components are frequently included in enjoyable physical activities. Teens are more likely to look forward to exercising when they connect with others, whether it be through team sports or group sessions.

2. Encouraging Regular Physical Activity Aligned with Interests

Promoting Frequent Exercise in Line with Interests: Techniques for Managing Adolescent Obesity

Teens who are obese frequently experience difficulties when they try to exercise regularly. The secret is to match their interests and preferences with activities that will make exercising more pleasurable and long-lasting.

This method acknowledges the need of customizing workout regimens to each person's interests in order to make fitness a pleasurable and long-lasting aspect of their lifestyle.

The following are some methods to help kids find regular physical activity that suits their interests:

1. Evaluate Interests and Preferences: To begin, have open-ended discussions with teenagers regarding their interests, passions, and favorite pastimes. This makes it easier to see possible integrations of physical activity with their current interests.

Examine their likes and personality. Which activities—individual or group—do they prefer? Workouts at a high or low intensity? Interior or outside settings? Knowing their preferences makes it easier to select appropriate solutions.

Think about their aptitudes and capabilities. In order to give them confidence and drive to keep going, encourage them to try things they are already skilled at or are interested in learning.

2. Provide a Variety of Activity Options: Go beyond conventional sports and fitness regimens. Investigate a variety of pursuits, such as rock climbing, biking, hiking, martial arts, yoga, swimming, rock climbing, and even motion-based video games.

Introduce engaging and novel activities. Look at popular exercise regimens, outdoor pursuits, or unusual activities that they may not have previously thought about.

Give people access to a range of resources. Urge them to look into fitness centres, parks, community centres, and internet resources that provide a variety of activities.

3. Encourage Trial and Discovery: Provide chances to try out various activities without committing to a long-term schedule. This enables teenagers to find interests, hidden talents, and activities they truly enjoy.

To lower potential cost obstacles and promote exploration, arrange free trial classes or introductory sessions in activities they indicate interest in.

Assist teenagers in finding the ideal fit for their interests and skills by partnering with teachers or fitness professionals who can lead them through a variety of activities.

4. Promote Social Interaction and Support: Inspire team sports or group activities. This increases the enjoyment and motivation of physical activity by fostering a sense of community, accountability, and shared experience.

Arrange fun, active get-togethers with loved ones. Along with being physically active, going on hikes, bike rides, or playing energetic games with one other encourages social contact and bonding.

Make connections between teenagers and wholesome role models who partake in interests-based activities. Observing people enjoying themselves while exercising can be motivating and motivational.

5. Use Technology and Gamification: Take a look at wearable technology, interactive games, and fitness applications that can enhance the fun and engagement of physical exercise. Particularly tempting to tech-savvy teenagers may be this.

To add a competitive element and encourage them to stay active, think about hosting online fitness challenges or virtual tournaments.

Make use of gamified fitness programmes and virtual reality experiences, which offer engaging and immersive methods to exercise.

6. Honor successes and forward motion:

No matter how long or how hard it lasts, acknowledge and enjoy any gain in physical activity. This encourages individuals to keep up their efforts and reinforces positive behavior.

Never compare yourself to others; instead, concentrate on your own growth and accomplishments. It also gives kids the confidence to set reasonable and doable goals by promoting a good self-image.

Give them little gifts of appreciation or enjoyable experiences in exchange for their hard work. They are given positive reinforcement and are inspired to maintain their motivation as they travel.

3. Prioritising Adequate Sleep for Improved Mood and Well-being

For the best possible physical and mental well-being, getting enough sleep is not merely a luxury. Prioritizing sleep is essential for teens facing the difficulties of adolescence in order to sustain positive mood, mental health, and cognitive function. Teens can experience better mood, increased cognitive performance, and overall well-being by prioritizing getting enough sleep and putting these ideas into practice. It is crucial to promote proper sleep patterns during adolescence because sleep, mood, and general health are all connected.

Teenagers need to prioritize sleep for the following reasons:

1. Better Mood and Less Anxiety: Getting enough sleep controls the release of chemicals like serotonin, which affect mood. Teens who get enough sleep are better able to handle stress and deal with difficult emotions.

These hormonal balances are upset by sleep deprivation, which exacerbates irritation, anxiety, and depressive symptoms.

Teenagers who prioritize their sleep are better able to handle the ups and downs of puberty and retain emotional stability.

2. Improved Cognitive Function and Academic Achievement: The brain forms new neural connections, absorbs information, and consolidates memories when we sleep. Teens who get enough sleep can wake up feeling focused and awake, ready to study and provide their best effort in the classroom.

Lack of sleep affects learning potential and academic performance by impairing memory, focus, and problem-solving skills.

Teenagers who prioritize their sleep are more rested and ready to learn with maximum cognitive performance.

3. Improved Physical wellness and Well-Being: Sleep is essential for immune system regulation and for fostering physical wellness.

Teens who get enough sleep are better able to heal from wounds, withstand illness, and have a balanced immune system.

Teenagers who lack sleep are more prone to infections and diseases because sleep loss impairs the immune system.

Teenagers who prioritize their sleep are better able to preserve their physical health and are shielded from future health issues.

4. Better Social Interactions and Relationships: Adolescents who get enough sleep exhibit more patience, empathy, and communication skills. Better social connections and stronger bonds with friends and family are fostered by this.

Lack of sleep can cause mood changes, impatience, and trouble controlling one's emotions. Relationships may suffer and social interactions may suffer as a result.

Teenagers who prioritize their sleep are better able to engage with others in a courteous and positive manner, which fosters supportive and healthy connections.

Teens can prioritize getting enough sleep by using the following strategies:

Even on the weekends, try your best to maintain a consistent sleep routine.

Establish a peaceful evening routine that involves soothing pursuits like music listening, warm baths, or reading.

Before going to bed, steer clear of sugary drinks and caffeine as these can disrupt your sleep.

For the best sleeping environment, make sure their bedroom is cold, quiet, and dark.

Don't spend too much time on screens right before bed because the blue light they create can interfere with your sleep.

Exercise on a regular basis, but try not to do it too soon before bed.

If your sleep issues don't go away, get expert assistance.

Teens can greatly enhance their mood, emotional well-being, cognitive performance, physical health, and social connections by prioritizing sleep and developing appropriate sleep patterns. This puts them on the right track for a happier and healthier future.

Chapter Five: Addressing Emotional Eating Patterns in Teen Obesity

The act of eating in response to negative emotions, or emotional eating, can pose a significant challenge for teens who struggle with obesity. While dietary habits and physical activity are still important, identifying and managing emotional eating patterns is equally important for long-term success.

The following is a comprehensive approach to addressing emotional eating in teens who struggle with obesity:

1. Identifying Emotional Triggers: Assist teens in identifying situations, emotions, and internal cues that set off their desire to eat for comfort; these could include stress, anxiety, boredom, sadness, or frustration. You can keep a food diary or track emotions and eating patterns to help identify specific emotional eating triggers and patterns. Encourage teens to discuss their feelings with one another and share their experiences with others.

2. Creating Healthy Coping Strategies: Find different ways to deal with unfavorable feelings. This could be physical activity, practicing calming methods like yoga or meditation, keeping a journal, conversing with friends or family, or taking up enjoyable hobbies.

Exercise your self-awareness and mindfulness. Encourage teenagers to identify their feelings and triggers before they turn to unhealthy coping techniques.

Provide a coping strategy toolkit that teenagers may easily access and apply to a variety of circumstances.

3. Changing Food and Drinking Routines:

Eat a diet rich in nutrients and balance. To avoid overindulging in food out of hunger, regularly provide access to wholesome foods and snacks.

Minimize processed foods, sugar-filled beverages, and unhealthy snack choices.

Cravings and emotional eating patterns may be influenced by these.

Promote mindful eating habits. Encourage teenagers to stop using food as a diversion and instead concentrate on the flavor, texture, and experience of eating.

Engage teenagers in the preparation and planning of meals. This encourages a feeling of control and ownership over their dietary decisions.

4. Seeking Professional Support: Take into account consulting a licensed therapist or dietitian for advice. They can offer tailored support and direction for forming wholesome eating habits and controlling emotional triggers.

In order to address the underlying familial dynamics that give rise to emotional eating patterns, family therapy sessions may be helpful.

Teens can interact and exchange experiences in a secure setting with others going through similar struggles in support groups.

5. Fostering Self-Compassion and a Positive Body Image: Promote acceptance and self-compassion. Encourage teenagers to avoid self-blame or judgment by helping them understand that emotional eating is a common coping method.

Adopt a body-positive and self-accepting mindset. Encourage teenagers to value their bodies for more than simply their appearance by spreading positive messages about good body image.

Honor advancements and non-scale victories. Prioritize total health, self-esteem, and emotional well-being over weight loss.

6. Creating a Supportive Network: Place friends and relatives in your teen's immediate vicinity. Promote candid communication and give them credit for their efforts.

Assist them in finding mentors or role models who can provide direction and encouragement based on their personal experiences.

Assist them in creating a network of people who support a healthy lifestyle choices and positive body image.

1. Identifying Emotional Triggers Leading to Unhealthy Eating Habits

Understanding the emotional causes that lead to harmful eating patterns in obese teens is essential to helping them develop good coping strategies and promoting their long-term health. Teenagers' connections with food are frequently greatly influenced by emotional issues.

We can assist kids in creating healthier connections with food by proactively recognizing and addressing the emotional triggers that result in harmful eating behaviors. A thorough strategy for addressing emotional triggers in teen obesity must include equipping them with coping mechanisms, encouraging candid communication, and attending to underlying emotional problems.

Significance of Emotional Triggers:

1. Emotional Eating Patterns: Stress, depression, or boredom can be managed with food in situations where emotional eating patterns are triggered.

2. Effect on Food Choices: Emotional moods have an impact on food choices, which frequently result in the consumption of comfort foods that are heavy in calories.

3. Coping Mechanisms: Eating disorders can be a coping mechanism for psychological discomfort, which can lead to the emergence or aggravation of obesity.

4. Loop of Emotional Eating: Unhealthy food choices are triggered by unpleasant emotions, which can result in a loop of emotional eating that causes guilt and further emotional pain.

Teens can be assisted in identifying their emotional triggers in the following ways:

1. Introspection and self-awareness:

Promote journaling: Urge teenagers to record their eating habits and feelings in a food journal. This can assist individuals in recognizing particular circumstances, feelings, and body language that set off their comfort-seeking eating need.

Directed introspection: Such as, "What emotions do you typically feel before you crave unhealthy foods?" or "What situations or events usually lead you to overeat?" are examples of open-ended inquiries. Deeper contemplation and self-discovery may result from this.

Exercises for mindfulness: Encourage teenagers to engage in mindfulness exercises, such as guided imagery or meditation, to help them become more conscious of their moods, thoughts, and physical sensations. This can assist them in identifying emotional cues before they result in unhealthful eating habits.

2. Recognizing typical triggers:

Stress and anxiety: When faced with familial difficulties, social anxiety, or academic pressure, many teenagers turn to emotional eating.

Boredom and loneliness: Teens who are socially isolated or lack stimulating activities may turn to food as a source of solace.

Sadness and frustration: Emotional eating can also be triggered as a coping mechanism by challenging emotions such as sadness, rage, or frustration.

Rewarding events and festivities: Overeating can occur when people associate food with happy occasions like holidays or birthdays.

Work with teenagers to pinpoint the precise feelings that lead to unhealthy eating. Interventions that are specifically designed to target particular emotional triggers are more effective.

3. Identifying bodily cues: Cravings: Strong desires for particular meals, particularly unhealthy ones, may indicate the presence of an emotional trigger.

Changes in appetite: Teenagers may feel that their hunger increases or decreases in reaction to certain emotions.

Physical discomfort: Teens who are experiencing emotional difficulty may turn to food as a coping mechanism for physical symptoms like headaches or upset stomachs.

4. Outside observations

Family relationships: Examine the eating habits and food-related communication styles of your family. Teenage emotional eating can be exacerbated by unhealthy food choices or stressful mealtime routines.

Social influence: Be mindful of how social media and peer pressure can encourage poor eating habits or issues with body image.

Environmental factors: Not having enough access to wholesome food options or being exposed to advertisements for junk food can also be triggers.

We can enable teenagers to create better coping strategies and make deliberate food choices by assisting them in identifying their emotional triggers. A critical first step on their path to a happy and healthy life is developing this self-awareness.

5. Identify Emotional States: Assist teenagers in identifying and categorizing their feelings. Understanding particular emotions can help one better understand what motivates harmful eating patterns.

6. Teach Stress Management Techniques: Explain methods for managing stress, like mindfulness, deep breathing, or exercise. Offering substitute coping strategies lessens the need to turn to food to cope with stress.

7. Address Root Causes: Look at possible causes of emotional triggers, such as interpersonal problems or stress at school. Teens can create more effective coping

mechanisms by addressing the underlying issues.

8. Promote a Positive Body Image: Encourage a self-esteem and positive body image. A better sense of self-worth lessens the probability of turning to food as a coping mechanism for unpleasant feelings.

9. Educate on Nutrition and the Value of Balanced Eating: Disseminate information on nutrition and the significance of eating a balanced diet. Making healthy food choices is made easier for teenagers when they are aware of how eating choices affect their general wellbeing.

10. Engage Mental Health Professionals: When dealing with intricate emotional triggers, mental health professionals should be consulted. Specialized interventions for emotional well-being can be obtained with mental health support.

11. Promote Well-Being Coping Mechanisms: Encourage the use of healthy, non-food coping mechanisms. Promoting a variety of coping strategies lessens the need to turn to food for emotional solace.

12. Offer Emotional Support: Encourage and offer emotional support. Adolescents can overcome emotional obstacles without turning to bad eating habits when they are in a supportive setting.

13. Family Involvement: Have conversations with families regarding coping strategies and emotional triggers. Fostering an environment of caring and reinforcing excellent behaviors are two benefits of family support.

Here are a few more pointers:

Assist teenagers in recognizing and expressing their feelings by using a "feelings chart" or other visual aids.

Encourage them to talk honestly and openly about their feelings and issues with overindulging in unhealthy foods.

Honor their accomplishments in recognizing triggers and creating effective coping strategies.

2. Developing Healthy Coping Mechanisms for Stress and Emotions

Effective stress and emotion management is essential for reducing emotional eating and boosting general well-being in youth who struggle with obesity. We give teens the tools they need to deal with stress and emotions in a healthy way by providing them with a wide range of healthy coping strategies. Promoting the use of these tactics contributes to a comprehensive strategy for addressing and preventing teen obesity while also promoting mental health.

Fostering positive mental health and avoiding dependency on bad eating habits need the development of appropriate coping mechanisms for stress and emotions.

The Value of Healthy Coping Strategies

1. Reducing Emotional Eating: To stop the loop of utilizing food as the main way to deal with stress or emotions, healthy coping strategies can be used as alternatives to emotional eating.

2. Resilience Building: Equipping teenagers with good coping strategies helps them become emotionally resilient, which makes it easier for them to deal with life's obstacles.

3. Long-Term Emotional Well-Being: Positive coping mechanisms help promote emotional well-being over the long term, which affects mental health in ways that go beyond the current adolescent issues.

The following techniques can assist teenagers in creating constructive coping strategies:

1. Recognizing coping mechanisms:

Assist teenagers in identifying their go-to coping strategies. Do they have any health issues? Do they really aid with stress management?

Examine a range of constructive coping mechanisms:

Moving around: Exercise lowers stress hormones and releases endorphins, which are organic mood enhancers. Encourage them to participate in sports, dance, yoga, or any other enjoyable activity. Promote consistent physical exercise as a way to reduce stress. Exercise releases endorphins, which have the dual benefits of improving mood naturally and giving stress relief.

Relaxation methods: Progressive muscle relaxation, guided visualization, deep breathing exercises, and mindfulness meditation can all help soothe the body and mind. Introduce deep breathing exercises, relaxation methods, and mindfulness practices. By lowering stress and fostering emotional regulation, these methods provide a more healthy way to deal with difficult emotions.

Creative expression: Expressing oneself creatively by writing, painting, drawing, or playing music can help people let go of their emotions and express themselves. Encourage creative endeavors like writing, music, and art. Teens can channel their emotions in a positive way through artistic expression, which promotes self-expression and self-discovery.

Social support: Teens can receive important support and learn good coping mechanisms for their feelings by talking to friends, family, or a therapist.

Hobbies: Getting involved in activities they enjoy, such as reading, gaming, or spending time outside, can help people unwind and feel good.

2. Creating a toolkit for coping: Help teenagers discover constructive coping techniques that suit them best. You can customize this "toolbox" to suit their requirements and tastes.

Develop your mastery of these coping strategies via practice. They become more adept at handling stress and emotions with regular practice.

Make coping mechanisms simple to get to. Promote the use of a journal, a phone app for relaxation, or the creation of a special area for activities that relieve stress.

3. Developing emotional intelligence and self-awareness:

Aid teenagers in recognizing and comprehending their feelings. Encourage them to verbalize their emotions rather than holding them inside.

Put your attention toward developing emotional intelligence. Teach them how to recognize the things that set off their emotions, control their reactions, and speak clearly.

Practice self-compassion and mindfulness. Encourage them to notice their feelings and thoughts in a thoughtful, judgment-free manner.

4. Establishing a supportive atmosphere: Make sure teens can share their feelings in a secure and encouraging environment without worrying about being judged.

Promote direct communication and attentive listening. Make them feel understood and heard.

Make connections for them with others who will be helpful. Someone who has similar experiences and coping mechanisms could be a buddy, mentor, therapist, or counselor.

Stress the value of having wholesome social relationships. During trying times, having a strong social network to lean on for companionship and emotional support is beneficial.

5. Celebrating accomplishments and advancements: Honor and applaud their efforts in creating and applying constructive coping strategies.

Give attention to their development rather than their flawless performance. Urge them to learn from their mistakes and to keep experimenting with different approaches until they discover the one that suits them the best.

Enable them to take charge of their feelings and welfare.

Through the development of constructive coping strategies, teenagers can effectively regulate their emotional reactions. As a result, they are less susceptible to emotional eating and have a positive relationship with food. Recall that mastering these abilities requires time and repetition, so continue to be understanding and encouraging of them as they progress.

Here are a few more pointers:

Urge anyone who is having trouble controlling their stress or emotions on their own to get professional assistance.

Encourage a balanced lifestyle that includes enough sleep, frequent exercise, and a nutritious diet.

Set a good example for others by using healthy coping techniques yourself.

1. Journaling and Self-Reflection: Promote journaling among teenagers as a means of introspection. Writing in a journal offers a private setting for managing feelings and understanding one's own experiences.

2. Effective Time Management and Organizational Skills: Instruct students in these areas. Improving these abilities fosters a sense of control by lowering stress associated with personal or academic obligations.

3. Use Cognitive Behavioral strategies: Reframe and confront unfavorable thought patterns by using cognitive behavioural strategies. More positive emotional reactions can be attributed to altered cognitive processes.

4. Healthy Sleep Habits: Stress the value of adhering to a regular sleep schedule. Resilience to stress and mental health are directly correlated with sleep quality.

5. Setting Boundaries: Stress the value of establishing sound boundaries in interpersonal interactions. Setting limits eases interpersonal dynamics-related stress and promotes emotional equilibrium.

6. Seeking Professional Support: Encourage seeking out professional mental health support when necessary. Experts can offer customized advice on creating coping strategies that meet specific needs.

7. Education on Nutrition and Its Effects: Disseminate information regarding the connection between mental health and nutrition. Knowing how food choices affect mood highlights how crucial it is to keep a balanced diet.

8. Fostering Positive Self-Talk: Encourage self-affirmations and positive self-talk. A

positive outlook and higher self-esteem are facilitated by positive affirmations.

9. Guided imagery and meditation: Explain the use of guided imagery and meditation techniques. These methods encourage calmness and have the potential to be useful in stress and mood management.

10. Promoting Healthy Interests and Hobbies: Encourage the growth of healthy interests and hobbies. Pleasurable hobbies offer a constructive way to release tension and feelings.

11. Family Involvement in Coping Strategies: Bring up coping strategies with families. Having supportive family members helps people adopt appropriate coping strategies.

3. Seeking Professional Guidance if Emotional Eating Patterns Persist

Even though self-awareness, constructive coping techniques, and encouraging surroundings can greatly enhance emotional eating patterns, in certain situations expert advice may be necessary for long-term success. This is the time when getting expert assistance is essential:

1. Persistent and Unmanageable Emotional Eating: See a professional if self-help techniques don't significantly improve emotional eating.

Professional assistance is required if the habits are interfering with day-to-day activities, producing a great deal of discomfort, or resulting in unhealthful weight fluctuations.

2. Co-occurring Mental Health issues: Trauma, anxiety, and depression are common mental health issues that co-occur with emotional eating.

For long-term emotional control and nutritious eating habits, treating these co-occurring disorders with a therapist or mental health specialist is crucial.

3. Difficulty Identifying and Managing Triggers: Some teenagers may find it difficult to recognize emotional triggers and to create useful coping techniques.

Expert advice can assist them in identifying their triggers, creating customized coping mechanisms, and resolving any underlying problems that may be causing them to overeat emotionally.

4. Unsupportive Environment or Family Dynamics: Emotional eating patterns may be influenced by social pressures, unhealthy family dynamics, or restricted access to healthful meals.

In order to address these outside influences and foster a more conducive atmosphere for good eating habits, seeking expert assistance can be helpful.

5. Lack of Progress or Relapses: Professional counsel can help identify and address any underlying issues preventing progress if, despite constant attempts, there is little progress or relapses repeatedly.

Additional help, accountability, and individualized solutions for overcoming obstacles can be obtained from a certified dietitian or therapist.

Different Forms of Expert Assistance:

A therapist or counselor can assist teenagers in developing coping skills, understanding their feelings, and taking care of any underlying mental health issues.

A registered dietitian can create nutritious meal plans, offer individualized nutrition counseling, and handle any dietary issues.

Family therapy: May assist in addressing communication styles and family dynamics that could be linked to emotional eating.

Advantages of Getting Professional Assistance:

-self-awareness and emotional control aree improved.

-creation of efficient coping strategies for emotions and stress.

-less susceptibility to bad eating habits and emotional eating.

-enhanced body image and sense of self-worth.

-more control over wellbeing and health.

Recall that asking for expert assistance is a show of strength and a desire to do better rather than weakness. Teens can obtain the tools and assistance they require to form wholesome eating habits, effectively regulate their emotions, and attain long-term wellbeing by completing this phase.

Chapter Six: Thriving Beyond Obesity

Adolescent obesity is a complicated problem with wide-ranging effects. Teenagers' entire well-being requires a holistic approach that addresses physical, emotional, and social elements in order to manage it effectively.

It is crucial to take a holistic approach to health, taking into account not only the physical aspects of well-being but also the emotional, social, and mental ones, in order to thrive beyond obesity. Adolescents can overcome the obstacles of obesity and thrive in all areas of their lives by adopting a holistic approach, paving the way for a future marked by resiliency, self-acceptance, and a lively sense of well-being.

This is a thorough approach for managing teens who are obese and beyond:

1. Encouraging body positivity and self-acceptance: Fight poor body image and use positive self-talk. Pay attention to your personal assets and inner attributes. Honor advancements and non-scale victories.

Establish a welcoming atmosphere that promotes acceptance and self-compassion.

2. Including Pleasurable Physical Activity: Find out what kids actually enjoy doing, as opposed to just what they consider to be "exercise." Provide a range of choices and encourage social engagement by organizing group activities. Prioritize progress over perfection and set reasonable goals. Honor accomplishments and promote enduring healthy behaviors.

3. Dealing with Emotional Eating Patterns: Assist teenagers in recognizing the emotional cues that result in unhealthful eating. Create healthy coping strategies to deal with stress and unpleasant feelings. Encourage self-awareness and mindfulness to help with emotional control. If you have significant emotional eating, get professional help.

4. Making Getting Enough Sleep a Priority for Your Best Health: Create a sleep-friendly environment and stick to a regular sleep routine. Limit your screen time before bed, stay away from sugary drinks and coffee.

Promote physical exercise, but refrain from working out right before bed. Acknowledge how critical sleep is to your physical, mental, and emotional well-being.

5. Creating a Supportive Network: Encircle teenagers with mentors, friends, and family who are upbeat and encourage making healthy decisions. Make connections for them with others who can provide direction and assistance..Promote open dialogue and establish a secure environment in which worries can be voiced. Encourage involvement in activities that provide a sense of community and social contact.

6. Professional Advice and Assistance: When in need, get assistance from therapists, certified dietitians, and other professionals. Take care of co-occurring mental health issues as they may be a factor in emotional eating. To address family dynamics that affect eating behaviors, use family therapy. Get access to tools and specialized programs created for obese teenagers.

7. Celebrating Success and Acknowledging
Progress: Pay attention to the process and
give credit for each effort made, no matter
how big or small. Celebrate your non-scale
successes, including better mood, more
energy, and healthier habits. Encouragement
and positive reinforcement can help to spur
on further development. Encourage
teenagers to take responsibility for their own
health and wellbeing.

We can enable adolescents who struggle with
obesity to flourish despite their weight by
putting these tactics into practice and
encouraging a comprehensive approach.
Recall that each person's journey is distinct,
and that continued understanding, support,
and dedication to their general well-being are
necessary for them to succeed.

1. Cultivating Self-confidence and Resilience in Teens: A Vital Aspect of Thriving Beyond Obesity

Resilience and self-assurance are crucial traits for teenagers overcoming adolescent obstacles. These attributes become even more important while managing obesity since they support good coping strategies, a positive self-image, and long-term success. Fostering resilience and self-assurance in teenagers is essential to helping them thrive beyond obesity and face obstacles head-on.

Adolescents who struggle with obesity can overcome health-related obstacles and lay a solid foundation for their future development by consciously fostering resilience and self-assurance. These attributes enable them to live genuinely beyond the limitations of obesity by embracing their journey with optimism, flexibility, and inner strength.

The Importance of Resilience and Self-Assurance:

1. Empowerment for good transformation: Adolescents with self-confidence are more able to accept their individuality and set out on a path toward good transformation.

2. Navigating Challenges: Teens who possess resilience are better able to handle obstacles and setbacks with fortitude and flexibility, which promotes a proactive attitude toward their wellbeing.

3. Good Self-Image: Developing self-assurance helps one have a positive self-image and a healthy relationship with their body.

4. Lifelong Skills: Resilience and self-assurance are lifelong traits that impact many facets of both personal and professional life after puberty.

Teens can develop resilience and self-confidence by implementing the following important strategies:

1. Self-awareness and Self-acceptance: Help teenagers reflect on their values, strengths, and distinctive characteristics.

Assist them in creating a good self-image that transcends their physical attributes, such as weight.

Encourage them to embrace their flaws and difficulties and to be compassionate with themselves.

2. Challenging Limiting Beliefs and Negative Thoughts: Give teenagers the skills they need to recognize and confront self-talk and negative thoughts.

Urge them to substitute self-encouragement and positive affirmations for negativity.

Encourage a growth mentality that places more value on effort, learning, and progress than on perfection.

3. Establishing Reachable Objectives and Honoring Achievements: Assist teenagers in establishing practical, reachable objectives that prioritize advancement over perfection.

No matter how minor the accomplishment, acknowledge each milestone.

Acknowledge and honor their hard work and dedication to the cause.

4. Creating Healthy Coping Mechanisms: Provide teenagers with a variety of coping skills to help them deal with stress, anxiety, and other unpleasant feelings.

Promote healthy outlets such as journaling, artistic expression, exercise, and relaxation methods.

Assist them in developing a toolkit of coping techniques they can use in various circumstances.

5. Creating a Supportive Network: Encircle teenagers with mentors, friends, and relatives who are upbeat and encouraging.

Urge them to make connections with people who have gone through comparable struggles or experiences.

Make sure kids can get in touch with experts like counselors or therapists when they need them.

6. Developing Resilience through Difficulties: Motivate teenagers to see obstacles and failures as chances for development.

Encourage them to persevere and adopt a "never give up" mentality.

Honor their capacity to overcome hindrances and recover from misfortune.

7. Encouraging Self-compassion and Positive Body Image: Resist peer pressure and unattainable beauty standards.

Urge teenagers to emphasize inner beauty and to value their bodies for what they can accomplish.

Encourage body-positive messaging and confront irrational assumptions.

8. Encouraging Advocacy and Self-expression in Teens:

Urge teenagers to speak out for their needs and for themselves.

Give them the chance to freely express their emotions and experiences.

Give them the freedom to engage in roles and activities that bolster their self-esteem and feeling of community.

We can give teenagers the inner power and positive self-image they need to thrive beyond obesity by encouraging resilience and self-confidence. These attributes will be invaluable to them throughout their lives, enabling them to overcome obstacles, accomplish their objectives, and lead happy, full lives.

2. Celebrating Non-scale Victories and Progress Markers

While controlling teen obesity frequently revolves around weight loss, it's important to acknowledge and appreciate non-scale successes and milestones along the way. Even seemingly insignificant accomplishments can have a big impact on motivation, foster a favorable self-image, and help pave the way for long-term success.

Teenagers are taught to acknowledge the complex nature of their journey towards well-being by actively recognizing non-scale achievements and progress markers. In the pursuit of health and living beyond obesity, cultivating a positive mindset surrounding accomplishments beyond numerical measures helps to preserve motivation, confidence, and a holistic sense of accomplishment.

Why Non-Scale Wins Are Important:

1. All-encompassing Well-being: Non-scale victories cover a range of well-being dimensions, such as physical, social, and emotional achievements.

2. Motivation and Confidence: Highlighting accomplishments strengthens one's resolve to pursue health objectives by increasing motivation and confidence.

3. Move from Numbers to Achievements: Emphasizing non-scale successes causes one to refocus on significant accomplishments rather than numerical measurements, which in turn fosters a more positive relationship with one's journey.

4. Sustainable Lifestyle Habits: Adopting sustainable lifestyle practices is a common indicator of non-scale successes and promotes long-term wellbeing.

The following are some main advantages of applauding non-scale successes:

1. Increased Motivation and Sustainability: Acknowledging accomplishments that go above and beyond the scale encourages positive behavior and gives people the will to keep moving forward. Teens who use it feel more in charge of their health and wellbeing and more powerful.

2. Better Body Image and Self-esteem: Highlighting non-scale successes helps people appreciate their bodies' capacities beyond weight and develop a positive self-image. It enables them to concentrate on development and personal improvement rather than merely the scale's number.

3. A greater sense of success: Teens who receive praise and recognition for their efforts, no matter how minor, feel more proud of their efforts and a sense of accomplishment. This encourages individuals to keep going on and supports their optimistic self-talk.

4. Fostering Resilience and Perseverance: Recalling prior successes and benchmarks can inspire individuals and fortify their determination to surmount obstacles when confronted with obstacles or disappointments.

Instances of Non-Scale Victories to Honor:

Enhanced vitality and better-quality sleep:
These signify improved general health and
wellness.

Increased confidence and enjoyment of
physical activities might result from having
more physical strength and endurance.

Better eating habits and more self-control:
These indicate a shift in lifestyle that will
last.

The development of good coping strategies
gives teenagers the ability to effectively
control their stress and emotions.

A change toward self-acceptance and
appreciation is shown by more positive
self-talk and body image.

Participating more in fun activities
encourages a sense of community and a
healthy lifestyle.

Improved friendships and family ties: These things add to general happiness and wellbeing.

Methods for Celebrating Non-Scale Victories:

Establish a "victory journal" to record advancements and successes.

Review and recognize your progress on a regular basis, no matter how tiny.

Reward achievements and hard work with little gestures of gratitude.

Celebrate your victories with dependable friends and family.

Share happy thoughts on your personal blog or on social media.

Take part in leisure and self-care-oriented pursuits.

Pay attention to the process rather than the end result.

By acknowledging and applauding non-scale successes, we can help teens on their path to a happy, healthy life. Regardless of height or weight, these successes are important indicators of their development and dedication to general well-being.

3. Embracing a Healthy Lifestyle as a Path to Overall Well-being

It is vital to adopt a healthy lifestyle as a means of achieving overall well-being in the context of managing teen obesity, rather than concentrating only on weight loss. Adopting a healthy lifestyle involves a transformative journey that encompasses mental, emotional, and social well-being in addition to physical health.

Beyond the numbers on the scale, long-term health advantages, pleasant self-image, and sustainable habits are emphasised in this comprehensive approach.

Adopting a healthy lifestyle is a comprehensive commitment to general well-being rather than only a set of behaviors. Individuals, particularly teenagers, can begin on a life-changing journey that includes physical health, mental clarity, emotional resilience, and social connection by implementing these tactics into their everyday lives. This will ultimately lead to a fulfilling and vibrant life.

The Significance of a Healthy Lifestyle in Its Whole:

1. Physical Health: A balanced lifestyle promotes the best possible physical health, which boosts immunity, longevity, and energy levels.

2. Mental Well-Being: Consistent exercise and a healthy diet have a beneficial effect on mental well-being by encouraging resilience, clarity, and attention.

3. Emotional Resilience: Living a healthy lifestyle helps people become emotionally resilient, which gives them useful coping skills for stressful situations.

4. Positive Self-Image: Developing a healthy lifestyle fosters a positive sense of self-worth and self-image, which in turn encourages self-acceptance and self-assurance.

5. Social Connection: Maintaining a healthy lifestyle and engaging in shared activities can fortify social relationships and provide a network of support.

6. Disease Prevention: Adopting a healthy lifestyle is essential for preventing chronic illnesses and promoting long-term wellbeing.

The following are essential elements in adopting a healthy lifestyle:

1. Balanced Diet: Emphasize complete, unprocessed foods high in whole grains, fruits, vegetables, and lean protein.

Promote sensible eating habits and sensible portion amounts.

Limit processed snacks, sugar-filled beverages, and unhealthy fats.

Involve teenagers in meal preparation and planning to encourage self-sufficiency and healthy choices.

2. Frequent Exercise: Look for fun and interesting hobbies besides athletics.

To provide support and motivation, promote social interaction and group activities.

To stay motivated, keep your attention on small steps and acknowledge your accomplishments.

Include exercise in your everyday routine to ensure long-term sustainability.

3. Sufficient Sleep: Make sure you prioritize proper sleep hygiene and create a regular sleep regimen.

Establish a calming nighttime ritual and cut down on screen time before bed.

To help you sleep better, practice mindfulness and relaxation practices.

Acknowledge the significance of sleep for both mental and physical well-being.

4. Emotional Well-Being: Create constructive coping strategies to deal with stress, worry, and other unpleasant feelings.

Develop self-awareness and good communication techniques to convey emotions.

To increase self-esteem, encourage self-compassion and encouraging self-talk.

When necessary, get professional assistance to manage mental health issues.

5. Positive Social Support: Give teenagers mentors who promote healthy choices, as well as friends and family who are there to support them.

Create a robust social network that fosters a sense of identity and well-being.

Promote candid dialogue and establish a secure environment for discussing difficulties.

Employ support networks for additional support and guidance.

6. Mindfulness and Self-Care: To reduce stress and foster relaxation, promote techniques like yoga, meditation, and journaling.

Place a focus on self-care practices that enhance contentment and overall health.

Promote interests and pastimes that make you happy and fulfilled.

Encourage a sense of direction and self-worth that goes beyond looks.

Teens can transcend obesity and attain long-term well-being by adopting a healthy lifestyle. This strategy focuses on holistic health, a good self-image, and a long-term strategy for leading a healthy lifestyle rather than just weight loss. Recall that the goal of the journey is progress rather than perfection, and that long-term success depends on appreciating each accomplishment as it is made.

Chapter Seven: Practical Guidance for Managing Teen Obesity

Teenage obesity management calls for a comprehensive strategy that takes into account social, emotional, and physical factors. This all-encompassing approach takes into account lifestyle, mental, and physical health aspects in addition to physical health, creating an atmosphere that is both supportive and long-lasting for kids as they work toward better overall health.

The following useful actions can help families, teenagers, and medical professionals:

For teenagers:

1. Motivation and self-awareness:

Maintain a food journal: Monitor your intake of food, your mood, and your physical activity to find trends and triggers.

Establish reasonable objectives: Pay attention to small steps and acknowledge non-quantitative achievements such as more energy or happier mood.

Determine constructive coping strategies: To control your stress and emotions, engage in mindfulness exercises, relaxation methods, or pastimes.

Develop compassion for yourself: Adopt an optimistic mindset and acknowledge failures as teaching moments.

2. Eating practices that promote health: Give complete, unprocessed foods priority. Make your choice of lean protein, whole grains, fruits, and vegetables.

Together, plan and cook the meals: This fosters ownership and participation in making good decisions.

Limit processed snacks and sugar-filled beverages: Choose water and wholesome substitutes.

Eat mindfully by paying attention to flavor, texture, and hunger signals to prevent overindulging.

3. Frequent exercise:

Look for fun things to do: Take up dancing, yoga, athletics, or whatever else they find enjoyable.

Start out slowly and build up your intensity over time: Make it a habit and concentrate on being consistent.

Include exercise in your everyday routine by walking, climbing stairs, or actively doing housework.

Get a workout partner or participate in group activities: Motivation and accountability are increased by social engagement.

4. Sufficient sleep: Create a regular sleep schedule: Try to get 8–10 hours each night.

Establish a peaceful evening routine by reading, taking a warm bath, or listening to quiet music.

Limit your screen time before bed because the blue light that gadgets emit can interfere with your sleep.

Make sure your bedroom is cold, quiet, and dark because these factors encourage deeper sleep.

5. The state of mind:

Determine the feelings that lead to unhealthy eating: Identify the circumstances, feelings, or inner signals that trigger cravings.

Create healthy coping strategies by practicing deep breathing, writing in a notebook, talking to trustworthy people, or taking up a hobby.

Seek out expert assistance: In order to address underlying issues, contemplate treatment or counselling if emotional eating persists considerably.

Regarding Families:

Establish a warm environment by promoting transparent communication, refraining from criticism, and emphasizing rewards.

Set an example for others to follow: Set an example of good food and exercise for your kids.

Together, prepare wholesome meals: Make the family's dinner preparation a lively and enjoyable pastime.

Limit junk food and beverages when you're at home: Make sure there are plenty of healthy options available.

Rejoice at non-scale successes: Acknowledge and value advancements that go beyond mere weight reduction, such heightened vitality or enhanced self-worth.

Seek expert advice: Seek guidance and support from a qualified therapist or registered nutritionist.

Regarding Medical Professionals:

Make a thorough evaluation: Examine the teen's familial relationships, mental stability, and physical health.

Create a customized treatment strategy: Attend to each person's needs and objectives, emphasizing emotional support, healthy habits, and behavior adjustment.

Work together with families: Give families the knowledge and tools they need to support their teenagers.

Link teenagers to the right resources: Make use of licensed dietitians, therapists, support groups, or other appropriate experts.

Track developments and modify tactics as necessary: Monitor developments, spot obstacles, and modify the plan as necessary.

Encourage a welcoming and upbeat atmosphere: Give kids the tools they need to take control of their health, avoid stigmatizing weight, and concentrate on health outcomes.

1. Professional Support

Teenage obesity management calls for a complete plan that takes into account social, emotional, and physical factors. In order to provide direction, resources, and encouragement during this journey, professional help is essential.

Teens with obesity can be empowered to successfully manage their weight, enhance their general health and well-being, and succeed in the long run on their path to a satisfying and healthy life by receiving all-encompassing expert help.

1. Healthcare professionals' involvement

Healthcare Professionals' Role in the Management of Adolescent Obesity

Health care providers are essential in helping families and adolescents who are obese. Their knowledge and direction are very helpful in creating individualized treatment programs, dispensing resources and instruction, and keeping track of advancements. Healthcare practitioners can participate in the following important ways:

1. Assessment and diagnosis: Perform a thorough physical examination and evaluate the patient's medical history.

Analyze your dietary consumption and degree of physical activity.

Determine any co-occurring medical illnesses or issues with mental health.

Assess the degree of obesity and any associated health risks.

2. Development of treatment plans: Work together with families and teenagers to craft an individualised treatment plan.

Establish attainable objectives with a focus on healthy habits, behavior modification, and general well-being.

Encourage dietary changes and sensible eating practices.

Provide exercise regimens based on the requirements and preferences of each individual.

Make recommendations for counseling or therapy to address emotional and mental health issues.

3. Education and resources: Give families and teenagers evidence-based knowledge regarding appropriate weight management.

Provide teaching materials on healthy eating, exercise, and mental health.

Suggest self-help books, websites, or mobile applications to people who need further aid.

Make connections for them with local services such as weight management programs or support groups.

4. Observation and assessment:

Regularly monitor progress and evaluate how well the treatment plan is working.

Keep an eye on any weight loss, dietary modifications, and increases in physical activity.

Assess emotional and mental well-being.

Depending on the difficulties and advancements made, modify the therapy plan as necessary.

5. Cooperation and correspondence:

Work along with other medical specialists such as social workers, therapists, or registered dietitians.

To address concerns and offer assistance, keep lines of communication open with teenagers and their families.

Include families in the course of care to ensure consistency and support at home.

6. Advocacy and policy change: Push for laws and initiatives that encourage a healthy diet and regular exercise in local communities and schools.

Increase awareness of the problems associated with teen obesity and the requirement for all-encompassing support.

Work together with researchers to create and assess successful teen obesity therapies.

To effectively engage healthcare professionals, it is necessary to establish rapport and trust with teenagers and their families.

-emphasizing self-management and empowerment techniques.

-delivering inclusive, culturally aware care.

-keeping abreast with the most recent evidence-based procedures.

-working together with other experts to deliver complete care.

Through proactive involvement of healthcare professionals in managing teen obesity, we may establish a network of support that enables teenagers to reach their health and wellness objectives.

2. Teamwork-oriented methods

In order to effectively manage teen obesity, a team approach including many healthcare experts collaborating to help the adolescent and their family is necessary. Collaborative efforts guarantee all-encompassing treatment that tackles the psychological, social, and physical facets of obesity.

These are the main participants in a cooperative approach:

1. Primary Care Physician: Assessments and diagnoses patients initially.

-keeps an eye on general health and treats any co-occurring illnesses.

-plans the recommendations to other experts.

2. Registered Dietitian: Formulates individualized dietary programs according to each person's requirements and preferences.

-provides information on sensible portion sizes and eating habits.

-offers direction on controlling cravings and emotional eating.

3. Therapist or Counselor: Deals with emotional issues like stress, anxiety, or sadness that are linked to obesity.

-creates constructive coping strategies for handling stress and emotions.

-offers assistance for problems with self-esteem and body image.

4. Physical Activity Specialist: Crafts individualized fitness plans based on the teen's skills and preferences.

-tracks development and modifies the program as necessary.

-encourages engaging in physical activity as a pleasurable pastime.

5. Family Therapist: Deals with communication styles and family issues that could be linked to bad eating habits.

-helps families make good lifestyle choices by offering assistance.

-aids in providing a nurturing environment for the adolescent's wellbeing in homes.

Benefits of Collaborative Approaches:

-enhanced professional coordination and communication.

-thorough evaluation and a comprehensive plan of care that addresses every facet of obesity.

-enhanced support and accountability for the adolescent and their family.

-better availability of a wide range of resources and knowledge.

-increased drive and commitment to the prescribed course of care.

Elements of a Fruitful Collaboration:

Clearly stated roles for each professional and open communication.

Meetings and discussions on a regular basis
to talk about the difficulties and progress.

Unified aims and goals for the adolescent's
welfare.

Appreciation for the knowledge and efforts of
every professional.

Communicate honestly and openly with the
adolescent's family.

Collaborative model examples include:

Multispecialty clinics: Give comprehensive
treatment under one roof.

Platforms for telehealth: Enable expert
consultations virtually.

Programs centered around communities:
Provide workshops on healthy cooking,
fitness programs, and support groups.

Through promoting cooperation among
medical professionals, we may establish a
thorough and encouraging atmosphere that

enables obese youth to adopt healthy lifestyle choices and lead long, fulfilling lives.

2. Sleep Hygiene

1. Recognizing the Significance of Sleep for Obese Teens

A vital component of general health and wellbeing is sleep, particularly for obese teenagers. Our bodies heal wounds, balance hormones, and solidify memories as we sleep. Teens who are obese, however, frequently have sleep problems, which can lead to a vicious cycle of weight increase and health issues.

Teens with obesity can enhance their physical and mental well-being, aid in weight control, and achieve long-term well-being by realizing the significance of sleep and making healthy sleep habits a priority.

Teens that are obese need to sleep because of the following reasons:

1. Controls hormones: Hormones like ghrelin, which causes feelings of hunger, and leptin, which causes feelings of fullness, are produced in large quantities when people sleep. This equilibrium is upset by sleep deprivation, which increases appetite and creates desires for unhealthy foods, which ultimately results in weight gain.

2. Enhances metabolism: The mechanism by which your body burns calories for energy is known as metabolism, and it is greatly influenced by deep sleep. Insufficient sleep causes the metabolism to slow down, which makes it more difficult to keep a healthy weight.

3. Reduces inflammation: Lack of sleep causes the body to react inflammatory, which has been related to a number of diseases, including diabetes and cardiovascular disease, which are frequent co-morbidities with obesity.

4. Reduces stress hormones: Prolonged stress raises cortisol levels, a hormone that encourages fat storage, which may lead to obesity. Getting enough sleep lowers stress levels, which helps with cortisol surge prevention and weight management.

5. Enhances cognitive function: Lack of sleep has a detrimental effect on cognition, which can cause issues with focus, remembering, and making wise decisions. This may make it more difficult to stay motivated and follow diet recommendations.

6. Improves mood and mental health: Inadequate sleep is linked to a higher chance of anxiety and despair, which can result in unhealthy coping strategies like emotional eating. Getting enough sleep helps you feel happy and stable, which supports appropriate weight management.

7. Improves physical performance: Getting enough sleep is critical for the growth and repair of muscles, as well as for physical activity and fitness, both of which are critical for managing weight. Strength, endurance,

and general physical performance are all enhanced by getting enough sleep.

2. Creating wholesome sleeping schedules

Developing Healthful Sleep Schedules for Obese Teens

Teens who struggle with obesity must establish and stick to proper sleep habits in order to maximize their general health and wellbeing. The following are some essential tactics to promote restful sleep:

Establish a Regular Sleep Schedule: Even on weekends, go to bed and wake up at the same time every day. This aids in maintaining the normal sleep-wake cycle of your body.

Adolescents should have realistic bedtime and wake-up timings that accommodate 8–10 hours of sleep per night.

2. Create a Calm Bedtime Routine: Create a peaceful nighttime ritual, such as reading a book, having a warm bath, or listening to music that promotes relaxation. Steer clear

of mentally taxing activities like watching TV or using electronics.

Create a dark, quiet, and cool sleep environment.

3. Reduce Screen Time Before Bed: The hormone melatonin, which is essential for sleep, is suppressed by the blue light that electronic gadgets emit. Give yourself at least an hour before bed to avoid using screens.

Think about charging electronics outside of the bedroom to cut down on temptation and establish a sleep-friendly atmosphere.

4. Exercise Regularly: Physical activity on a regular basis improves the quality of sleep; however, avoid intense exercise right before bed. On most days of the week, try to get in at least 30 minutes of moderate-intensity exercise.

5. Manage Stress and Anxiety: Create healthy coping strategies to deal with stress and anxiety, such as journaling, deep

breathing exercises, or relaxation techniques.

Take care of any underlying mental health issues that might be causing your sleep problems.

6. Steer clear of alcohol and caffeine: Caffeine can disrupt sleep, so cut back on your intake, particularly in the afternoon and evening.

Alcohol should not be consumed right before bed because it can cause sleep disruptions and fragmentation.

7. Encourage Healthful Eating Practices: Keep a well-balanced diet full of healthy grains, fruits, vegetables, and lean protein. Aim to avoid large meals and sugary snacks right before bed.

Your body's internal clock can be regulated and improved sleep can be encouraged with regular meal times.

8. Seek Professional Assistance if Needed:
Speak with your healthcare professional if
your sleep problems don't go away after
trying these solutions. They are able to rule
out any underlying illnesses and suggest
different courses of action.

Teens who struggle with obesity can enhance
their quality of sleep and overall well-being
by adopting these habits into their daily
lives.

Chapter Eight: Empowering Families in the Management of Teen Obesity

Families are extremely important in helping obese teenagers. Families may inspire their teenagers to make healthy decisions, embrace sustainable lifestyle changes, and attain long-term well-being by creating a pleasant and encouraging atmosphere.

The following are some essential tactics that families can use to empower their obese teenagers:

1. Establish a Helpful Environment:

Steer clear of criticism and concentrate on offering praise.

To comprehend the difficulties and worries that your kid is facing, engage in open communication and active listening.

Celebrate improvements and successes of all sizes.

Show acceptance and love without conditions, irrespective of size or look.

2. Set an Example of good Behaviors: As a family, practice regular physical activity and good nutrition.

Plan and prepare meals with your teen and cook healthful meals together.

Take part in activities that you all enjoy, such as walking, playing sports, or dancing, to make physical activity fun.

Keep your body image positive and refrain from using language that disparages it.

3. Establish sensible objectives and acknowledge non-scale successes:

Set SMART (specific, measurable, achievable, relevant, and time-bound) goals with your adolescent together.

Prioritize development over weight loss. Celebrate your non-scale successes, like as better mood, more energy, and healthy food or exercise habits.

Establish a "victory journal" to record advancements and accomplishments while offering inspiration and support.

4. Promote Open Communication and Problem-Solving: Provide a secure environment where your adolescent can voice their emotions and worries without fear of repercussions.

Assist your teen in identifying the things that lead to unhealthy eating and in creating constructive coping strategies.

Collaborate to overcome obstacles and come up with ideas that will benefit your family.

If necessary, get professional assistance from a therapist or counsellor to deal with any underlying emotional problems.

5. Create a Support System: Use internet forums or support groups to get in touch with other families going through comparable struggles.

Encourage your adolescent to engage in enjoyable activities and form wholesome bonds with peers who endorse their healthy living choices.

Consult with medical doctors, registered dietitians, or physical activity specialists for advice and assistance.

6. Encourage Body Positivity and Self-Compassion: Assist your adolescent in cultivating positive self-talk and self-compassion.

Encourage body-positive messaging and question arbitrary notions of beauty.

Encourage your adolescent to place more emphasis on their skills and talents than just their size or look.

Assist children in developing a positive connection with food and exercise, and in appreciating the capabilities of their bodies.

7. Respect Individuality and Preferences: Adolescents are distinct individuals who could have various needs and preferences.

Instead of comparing your adolescent to other people, pay attention to their own development and adventure.

Be adaptable and ready to change your strategy in response to your teen's demands and input.

8. Make it Fun and Engrossing: Pay attention to how to make healthy decisions interesting and pleasurable.

Include enjoyable activities in your everyday routine, such as exploring the outdoors, attempting new sports, or preparing healthful meals together.

Make healthy living a family affair and spend quality time together doing things that are good for you.

Families may encourage their obese teens to take charge of their health and well-being by putting these recommendations into practice. Recall that this path calls for cooperation, tolerance, and patience. Families may foster a healthy and encouraging atmosphere that enables adolescents with obesity to flourish and reach their full potential by cooperating as a unit and asking for help when necessary.

1. Involving Parents and Caregivers in Teen Obesity Management

In order to properly manage teen obesity, parental and caregiver engagement is essential. Their guidance, compassion, and support can make a big difference in their teen's path to a happy, healthy life.

Involving parents and other caregivers has the following major advantages:

1. Enhanced motivation and treatment plan adherence: Teens are more likely to follow treatment programs and healthy habits when their parents are involved, which improves outcomes.

2. Better understanding and communication: Honest dialogue between parents and teenagers encourages cooperation and

understanding throughout the weight-management process.

3. Positive alterations to the home environment: To support their teen's healthy choices, parents can make positive alterations to the home environment, such as providing healthy food alternatives and promoting physical exercise.

4. Less stress and anxiety: Teens who receive parental support are better able to control their stress and anxiety levels, which can help them avoid bad eating habits.

5. Improved body image and self-esteem: Parents' encouragement and positive reinforcement can help adolescents develop a positive body image and increase their sense of self-worth.

Parental and caregiver involvement
strategies:

1. Raising awareness and educating parents:
Inform parents about the relationship
between mental health, physical activity,
good eating, and obesity in youth.

2. Collaboration and communication: Foster
frank dialogue about needs, difficulties, and
goals between parents and teenagers. Work
together to establish goals and treatment
regimens.

3. Provide parents with opportunities to
network, exchange experiences, and get
advice by hosting support groups and
workshops.

4. The fourth strategy is to use family-based
therapies, which deal with unhealthy eating
habits, communication styles, and family
dynamics inside the household.

5. Role modeling: Motivate parents to set an
example of good health by eating well,
exercising, and using constructive self-talk.

6. Positive reinforcement: To keep teens and parents motivated and committed, acknowledge their accomplishments.

7. Professional support: Instruct parents to consult therapists, certified dietitians, or healthcare professionals for advice if necessary.

8. Honoring individual needs: Admit that every family and adolescent has particular requirements and preferences. Adapt assistance and interventions to the unique circumstances of each family.

We can build a network of support that enables teenagers to make healthy choices and attain long-term health and well-being by actively integrating parents and caregivers in the management of teen obesity.

2. Creating a Supportive Environment

Fostering a supportive environment is crucial to assisting obese kids in reaching their health and wellness objectives. This involves creating a safe and supportive environment where teenagers feel empowered to make wise decisions and flourish, which goes beyond just offering wholesome food and promoting physical activity.

The following are essential components to establish a nurturing atmosphere:

1. Clear Communication and Help with Emotions:

Encourage frank and open dialogue about emotions, obstacles, and worries with weight and body image.

Give everyone your undivided love and acceptance, regardless of appearance or weight.

Be a judgment-free active listener and give your teen's feelings validation.

Throughout their journey, offer them encouragement and emotional support.

2. Positive Body Image and Self-Compassion: Encourage body positivity

and push back against unattainable beauty standards.

Encourage them to accept their bodies and to be kind to themselves.

Pay attention to their good traits and strengths rather than merely their weight.

Assist them in creating constructive coping strategies to deal with their negative self-talk.

3. Healthy Eating Practices: Make wholesome, well-balanced meals and snacks available.

Minimize sugar-filled beverages, processed foods, and harmful fats.

Promote attentive eating and put the enjoyment of food front and center.

Involve teenagers in meal preparation and planning to help them take responsibility for their dietary decisions.

4. Frequent Physical Activity: Promote engagement in enjoyable activities such as sports, dancing, or outdoor pursuits.

Make engaging in physical activity a pleasant family or group activity.

Pay attention to small steps forward and acknowledge accomplishments rather than just weight loss.

Assist them in locating activities that suit their interests and skill levels.

5. Cooperation and Goal-Setting: Work with your adolescent to create attainable and reasonable goals.

Prioritize long-term health behaviors over temporary cures.

Honor non-scale successes and recognize their advancement.

Cooperate with medical professionals and other networks of assistance.

6. Stress Management: Assist your adolescent in recognizing and controlling stressors.

Promote healthy coping strategies such as physical activity, mindfulness practices, or interests.

Give people the chance to express themselves freely and receive emotional support.

Take care of any underlying melancholy or worry that might be causing the poor eating.

7. Reduce Screen Time and Encourage Sleep: To encourage sound sleeping practices, reduce the amount of time spent on screens before bed.

Establish a calm, dark, and cool environment that promotes sleep.

Teens need eight to ten hours of sleep per night to perform at their best.

Avoid having large meals right before bed and cut back on coffee.

8. Reduce Stigma and Discrimination: Be sympathetic and enlightening while addressing stigma and discrimination related to weight.

Encourage acceptance and diversity in your household and neighborhood.

Dispel unfavorable myths regarding body image and weight.

Encourage your adolescent to confront weight bias and speak up for themselves.

Recall that fostering a supportive environment is an ongoing endeavor. Be understanding, accommodating, and patient. No matter how tiny, acknowledge your teen's accomplishments and continue to provide support and encouragement. As a team, you may foster an environment that encourages your adolescent to develop healthy behaviors, reach their full potential, and lead a happy and meaningful life.

Conclusion

1. Recap of key points:

Teenage obesity is a complicated problem that needs to be managed in many ways. This entails taking care of the social, emotional, and physical elements.

Experts are essential in offering direction, materials, and assistance. Collaboration between therapists, dietitians, physical activity specialists, and healthcare practitioners is required for this.

In order to create a nurturing environment, families are crucial. This entails encouraging candid dialogue, offering consolation, and setting an example of good behavior.

The secret to long-term success is empowering teenagers. Setting reasonable objectives, appreciating non-scale successes, cultivating self-compassion, and emphasizing a good body image are all necessary for this.

For general wellbeing, good sleep hygiene, stress reduction, and screen time moderation are crucial.

2. Motivation for sustained lifestyle

Modifications: Keep in mind that this is a journey, not a destination. There will be difficulties and disappointments, but keep going.

Prioritize progress over perfection. No matter how little a step you take toward your goals, remember to celebrate it.

Create long-lasting, health-conscious habits. Make incremental, tiny adjustments that work with your way of living.

Make time for the things you enjoy doing on a daily basis. You'll be more inclined to stick with them in the long run if you do this.

Never hesitate to seek for assistance. You can find a lot of materials to help you along the way.

3. Aspiring to a Healthier Future for Obese Teens

Notwithstanding the difficulties posed by teen obesity, there is a great deal of promise for a healthy future. This upbeat perspective is influenced by multiple factors:

1. Raising Knowledge and Inquiry:

Education programs and public awareness efforts are lowering stigma associated with obesity and fostering understanding of the condition.

Comprehensive health education programs that cover physical activity, nutrition, and body image are being implemented into schools.

The way that diversity and inclusivity are portrayed in the media is questioning unattainable beauty standards and encouraging positive body image.

2. Expanding Support Networks: To deliver comprehensive and individualised treatment,

collaborative healthcare models are bringing together a range of specialists.

Community-based initiatives promote a feeling of encouragement and belonging by providing workshops on healthy cuisine, fitness activities, and support groups.

Platforms for telehealth increase accessibility and convenience by giving users access to resources and expertise.

3. Innovative Interventions: To meet the specific needs of teenagers, researchers are creating and evaluating efficient interventions.

The primary goals of these therapies are skill development, behavior modification, and addressing underlying social and emotional issues.

Applications and solutions based on technology are being used to monitor progress, encourage healthy habits, and offer individualized support.

4. Put an emphasis on Prevention: To stop obesity before it starts, public health programs target young children and adolescents.

Healthy food choices and physical activity during the school day are encouraged by school lunch programs.

Entire neighborhoods are working to create accessible parks and safe routes for bicyclists and pedestrians to make good decisions.

5. Changing Cultural Narratives: A burgeoning body positivity and self-acceptance movement is encouraging varied body shapes and challenging unattainable beauty standards.

Positive messages about healthy living and weight Inclusivity are disseminated via social media platforms.

More and more influencers and celebrities are fighting the stigma associated with obesity and advocating for healthy lives.

6. Empowering Teens: The younger generation is actively participating in the health and well-being advocacy process.

To exchange stories and provide assistance, they are forming online forums and support groups.

They are speaking out in favor of improved access to healthcare, wholesome food options, and initiatives that encourage physical exercise.

7. Technological Developments: Customized tools for goal-setting, progress tracking, and motivation are now available through wearable technologies and smartphone apps.

Engaging and immersive worlds are being created using virtual reality experiences to encourage healthy behaviors and physical activity.

Customized treatments and on-demand support are being developed with the help of artificial intelligence.

The management of teen obesity appears to have a bright future thanks to these developing trends. Through the integration of enhanced consciousness, all-encompassing assistance networks, creative solutions, prophylactic actions, and constructive societal transformations, we may establish a society in which every adolescent has the chance to prosper and attain ideal health and wellness.

It's critical to keep in mind that sustained dedication and cooperation are needed to achieve this promising future. All of us have a responsibility to encourage healthy living, combat stigma, and offer assistance to young people who are struggling with obesity. By working together, we can build a more promising future where all young people have the confidence to lead healthy, happy lives.

For overweight teenagers, the future looks promising. With more investigation, instruction, and understanding, we can assist them in creating a healthier for themselves and generations to come.